GASTRIC SLEEVE

Healthy and Delicious Recipes for You to Enjoy After Weight Loss Surgery

(Healthy Cookbook After Gastric Sleeve Surgery for Weight Loss)

Candida Warfel

Published by Sharon Lohan

© **Candida Warfel**

All Rights Reserved

Gastric Sleeve: Healthy and Delicious Recipes for You to Enjoy After Weight Loss Surgery (Healthy Cookbook After Gastric Sleeve Surgery for Weight Loss)

ISBN 978-1-990334-86-3

All rights reserved. No part of this guide may be reproduced in any form without permission in writing from the publisher except in the case of brief quotations embodied in critical articles or reviews.

Legal & Disclaimer

The information contained in this book is not designed to replace or take the place of any form of medicine or professional medical advice. The information in this book has been provided for educational and entertainment purposes only.

The information contained in this book has been compiled from sources deemed reliable, and it is accurate to the best of the Author's knowledge; however, the Author cannot guarantee its accuracy and validity and cannot be held liable for any errors or omissions. Changes are periodically made to this book. You must consult your doctor or get professional medical advice before using any of the suggested remedies, techniques, or information in this book.

Table of contents

Part 1 1
Introduction 2
Gastric Sleeve Surgery Diet 5
Week 1: Clear liquid diet 5
Week 2: Full liquid diet 6
Week 3: Pureed food 7
Weeks 4-5: Soft food 8
Week 6 Onwards: Regular food 9
Chapter 1: The Liquid Diet and Sample Meal Plans 14
Week 1: Clear Liquid Diet 20
Week 2: Liquid Diet 22
Week 3: Pureed Food 25
Weeks 4 to 5: Soft Food 29
Week 6 Onwards: Solid Food 32
Chapter 2: Soft Food Recipes 35
Soft Food Preparation 37
Poultry Dishes 38
Scrambled Eggs With Pureed Kale and Cheese 38
Egg Drop Soup 40
Pork and Beef Dishes 42
Split Pea and Ham Soup 42
Classic Meatloaf 45
Texas Hash 48

Fish and Seafood Dishes 50
Parmesan Herb Crusted Baked Salmon 50
Lemon Garlic Tilapia 52
Vegetarian Dishes 54
Creamy Garlic Herb Mashed Potatoes 54
Dairy-Free Cheesy Zucchini Rice 56
Chickpea Salad 58
Chapter 3: Solid Food Recipes—Breakfast 60
Vegetarian Dishes 60
Pumpkin Bread 60
Vegan Vanilla Buttermilk Pancakes With Cinnamon 62
Cinnamon Swirl Loaf 64
Lemon and Poppy Seed Loaf 66
Pumpkin Pie Oatmeal 68
Non-Vegetarian Dishes 70
Blueberry and Cottage Cheese Pancakes 70
Denver Omelette 72
Spanish Tortilla with Ham 74
Fruity Yogurt Popsicles 76
Peanut Butter and Jelly Pancakes 77
Chapter 4: Solid Food Recipes—Lunch 78
Poultry Dishes 78
Cheesy Chicken Enchilada Soup 78
Cream of Chicken Soup 81
Avocado Egg Salad 83

Pork and Beef Dishes 85
Pulled Pork 85
Asian Pork Tenderloin 89
Fish and Seafood Dishes 91
Avocado Tuna Salad Sandwich 91
Apple and Tuna Sandwich 93
Vegetarian Dishes 94
Roasted Garlic Potato Soup 94
Tomato Soup 96
Tomato, Basil, and Quinoa Salad With Vegan Mozzarella 98
Chapter 5: Solid Food Recipes–Dinner 100
Poultry Dishes 100
Couscous Chicken Soup 100
Chicken with Peanut Applesauce 102
Baked Chicken and Vegetables 103
Pork and Beef Dishes 104
Shepherd's Pie 104
Pork and Black Bean Stew 106
Fish and Seafood Dishes 108
Pan-Fried Trout 108
Shrimp Ceviche 110
Vegetarian Dishes 111
Vegetarian Fried Rice 111
Roasted Root Vegetables 113
Vegetarian Chili 115

Chapter 6: Solid Food Recipes–Snacks, Sides, Desserts..117

Snacks 118

Cheesy Potato and Turkey Pancakes 118

Quinoa Fruit Salad With Honey Lemon Dressing........... 120

Apple Zucchini Bread.. 122

Blueberry Sour Cream Cake... 124

Sides 126

Mashed Cauliflower and Sweet Potatoes 126

Ham and Egg Baked Potato Bowls 128

Cauliflower and Cheddar Cheese Bake 130

Desserts 132

Apple Carrot Bread... 132

Vanilla Mug Cake... 135

Sticky Lemon Cake 137

Chapter 7: Tips When Dining Out 139

Chapter 8: How to Maintain Your Weight After Surgery 142

Establishing Healthy Eating Habits.................................. 142

Eat to Lose Weight 142

Meal Planning Is One of the Keys to Success 143

What Should You Be Eating? 143

Vitamins and Supplements... 145

Keep a Food Journal 145

Listen to Your Body 148

Be Mindful of Your Eating... 148

Be More Aware of Your Body 151

Physical Activity, Rest, and Dealing With Stress 152
Physical Activity 152
Managing Stress 156
Tracking Your Progress 158
Measurements and Photos 158
Changes in Your Home 159
Prepping Your Home 159
Shopping for Food 160
Items to Purchase Pre- and Post-Surgery 161
Your Support System 162
Family and Friends 162
Bariatric Medical Team 163
Part 2 166
Introduction 167
Chapter 1: Understanding Gastric Sleeve Surgery 168
Chapter 2: Gastric Sleeve Diet 171
Chapter 3: The Clear Liquids Diet 176
Chapter 4: Breakfast Recipes 177
Strawberry & Yogurt Smoothie Bowl 177
Blueberry & Veggies Smoothie Bowl 179
Warm Fruity & Cheese Bowl 180
Cheese & Yogurt Bowl 182
Banana Porridge 183
Pumpkin Porridge 184
Overnight Banana Oatmeal 186

Pumpkin & Cottage Cheese Oatmeal 187
Vanilla Crepes 189

Part 1

Introduction

A gastric sleeve surgery is a type of weight-loss surgery wherein 75-80% of a person's stomach is removed. This is also known as a Vertical Sleeve Gastrectomy. This is one of the more common bariatric procedures done. Out of all the bariatric surgeries done in the US, more than half of these are gastric sleeve surgeries, and the numbers increase every year (*Gastric Sleeve*, n.d.).

The patient needs to follow a diet that can help their surgery become a success. If your BMI is less than 50, start the diet two weeks before your surgery. If your BMI is greater than 50, start the diet four weeks before your surgery. Allot an additional three days for the liquid diet you need to be on before your surgery.

Following the pre-surgery diet for weight loss (*Bariatric Nutrition and Lifestyle Plan*, 2017):

•Helps reduce the fatty deposits around the liver, making it easier and safer for the surgeon to access the stomach.

•Promotes weight loss which lowers the risk of complications as obesity increases the risks of medical complications during surgery and post-op.

In addition, going through gastric sleeve surgery requires the patient to be committed to making changes in their lifestyle and their relationship with food. Following a pre-op diet helps the patient get started on changing their habits.

The pre-surgery diet should:

•Reduce calorie and carbohydrate intake. Protein intake should be increased. Trans Fats should be eliminated from the diet and there should be a focus on healthy fats. There are programs that recommend reducing calorie intake to 800 to 1,200 per day.

- Drink lots of water. Try to eliminate sodas and alcoholic beverages from your diet.

You may follow the 3 + 2 + 5 diet plan, which consists of:

- 3 protein shakes

- 2 low calorie entrees (each entree should just be 200 to 400 calories)

- 3 servings of non-starchy vegetables and 2 servings of fruits (no dried fruit or juice)

If you are still hungry, you may add another shake or another entree.

Make sure to eat breakfast within two hours of waking up and do not go more than 5 hours without eating. Doing this will increase your energy and let you lose weight. You may also start with your food journal during this time.

You can also start taking the vitamins and supplements when you start your diet. **Do not take iron and calcium supplements at the same time**. Take one with a 2 hour gap in between as iron restricts the absorption of calcium.

Drink 48 to 64 ounces of fluids everyday, preferably water.

Two to three days before the gastric sleeve surgery, the patient needs to switch to a purely liquid diet (but no soda is allowed). The patient needs to fast starting at midnight before surgery. Some medications, such as blood-thinning medication, arthritis medicine, herbal supplements, and nonsteroidal anti-inflammatory drugs should not be taken before surgery. It would be best to discuss your medications and supplements with your doctor with regards to discontinuing them before surgery.

Five millimeter incisions are made on the abdomen so small trocars can be inserted. A small camera is also inserted in the abdomen. An inspection of the stomach is done and blood vessels are divided. A Bougie tube is inserted into the stomach. This will provide the size of the stomach. The stomach is then surgically stapled into two, then removed, leaving around 20 to 25 percent of the original stomach. The portion of the stomach that has been removed produces the hormone ghrelin, which is a hunger-stimulating hormone, therefore making the patient experience hunger less often. This procedure takes about 40 to 70 minutes. Pain is manageable and doesn't require too much pain medication. Three to four hours after surgery, patients should be walking around. A stay of one or two nights at the hospital is required. In about two to four weeks, patients should be able to go back to school or work, although during the first two weeks, patients tend to feel more tired due to the liquid diet they have to be on. While there is reduced calorie intake during this time, most do not feel hungry. Four weeks after the procedure, patients can begin exercising (*Gastric Sleeve*, n.d.).

Because the stomach volume has been reduced, those who have undergone the surgery experience satiety faster, and food passes the stomach and intestines quicker. Also, the release of hunger hormones are reduced so people tend to feel less hungry. Those who undergo this surgery lose, on average, about 60 to 70 percent of excess weight, and reach their lowest weight a year or two after the surgery is done. There is an 80 to 90 percent success rate with gastric sleeve surgery.

Who are the suitable candidates for gastric sleeve surgery? Those who are considered:

- Have a body mass index (BMI) score of at least 40 *or* have a BMI of at least 35 and have other medical conditions that may be improved through weight loss, such as high blood pressure and type 2 diabetes.
- Are healthy enough to go through anesthesia and surgery.
- Have a commitment to weight loss and maintaining their weight loss after the surgery by changing their lifestyle and diet.
- Have tried losing weight through diet and exercise for at least six months and have not made any progress.

Gastric Sleeve Surgery Diet

It is important that the patient eases himself into the post-surgery diet to realize the benefits of the gastric sleeve surgery and also to avoid complications, such as gastric leaks, diarrhea, constipation, nausea, and vomiting.

Week 1: Clear liquid diet

A clear liquid is required so that your body can easily break it down and not put any strain on your digestive system. This type of diet does not provide sufficient nutrients to your body. Drink water, sugar-free versions of drink mixes such as Kool Aid, decaffeinated beverages, and clear broth.

The liquid should be at room temperature when consumed. Skip soda, drinks with caffeine, and beverages with added sugar.

You will start with a small amount, 1 fluid ounce, every hour every four hours, and increase by 1 fluid ounce after four hours.

Week 2: Full liquid diet

This includes items such as juice, protein shakes, milk, yogurt, and broth. You may also have sugar-free ice cream and pudding, cream of wheat, and applesauce. You need to separate your clear liquid intake with the full liquid meals. Wait an hour after drinking the full liquid meals to drink clear liquids.

You protein shakes should be low in sugar and calories; no more than 180 calories and 7 grams of sugar per serving. It should have at least 20 grams of protein. Your protein shake should not contain aspartame, but sucralose is acceptable.

The yogurt should be low calorie, low sugar, and high protein. It should have no more than 7 grams of sugar. It should not have added fruit, no added sugar, and no chunks. You may add flavored protein powder to your yogurt.

For the broths and soups, you may add unflavored protein powder. No noodles, grains, or rice with your soup or broth. The soup should not have chunks and should not have high fat cream. No chili, lentil, or bean soups.

Buy a variety of flavors as your tastes may change during this period. A good tip is to buy "base" flavors such as unflavored, vanilla, and chocolate protein powders, and then buy a variety of sugar-free syrups to enhance the protein shake. Same thing with your broth; you can buy chicken soup as your base, then enhance it with different herbs and spices. Do not use spicy seasonings, however, as these may not agree with your digestive system at this time.

Make it a habit to read the labels and nutrition information of your food. If you have any questions about your diet, contact your dietitian immediately.

Exercise should be no more than 10 minutes per session, and no more than half an hour each day. Start off slowly, but move often. Two weeks after your surgery, increase the duration every week until you're exercising for 30 to 45 minutes a day, five to seven days a week. Consult with your doctor and get cleared before you lift weights or go swimming.

Week 3: Pureed food

Stick to food such as cottage cheese, hummus, and other pureed foods. You need to separate your food intake with your fluid intake. Wait an hour after your food intake to drink any fluids.

Keep with your 30 to 45 minute, 5 to 7 days a week exercise regime.

Weeks 4-5: Soft food

Your calorie intake should be at 400 to 600 per day, with protein intake at 50 to 60 grams per day, or more if you can tolerate it. Eat three meals and one or two snacks each day, eating these at regular, scheduled times daily. Never go more than 5 waking hours without eating.

In this phase, you may have eggs, soft fruit, ground meats, cooked vegetables, beans, and fish.

Avoid starchy foods, processed carbohydrates, grains, and baked products such as bagels, breads, cakes, noodles, rice, and crackers. These types of food expand in your stomach and may cause blockage or pain. For the same reason, do not eat coconut bits or coconut flakes.

Avoid potted meats which are low in protein but high in fat.

Avoid food that can make you relapse to unhealthy eating habits such as refined carbs and grains, fatty and fried foods, foods high in sugar, and dry foods.

Do not eat nuts or popcorn, which are harder to digest.

Eat your food slowly, taking dime-sized bites and sipping your drink. Take at least 20 minutes to finish a meal. Eating slowly allows you to listen for your fullness cues, and avoid dumping syndrome and overeating. If you are not hungry yet, but it is time to eat, take a few bites of protein to keep your eating schedule.

Since it is important that you eat slowly, buy some warming plates or baby warmer trays to keep your food warm while you are eating.

Consume 48 to 64 ounces of fluid each day. Similar to the previous phases, avoid carbonated, high calorie, and caffeinated drinks.

Continue taking your vitamins and supplements, as well as the 30 to 45 minute, 5 to 7 days a week exercise regimen.

Continue with logging your food, fluids, and exercise in your food journal. Make sure you weigh and measure your food intake, not only so you can log it accurately in your journal, but ultimately to ensure you're getting enough of the protein and other nutrients you need to stay healthy.

Week 6 Onwards: Regular food

You can start eating regular food; however, bear in mind to eat small amounts at a time, and eat frequently. The past few phases should have taught you what food you can tolerate. Keep building on that and trying new foods. Continue with your healthy eating habits to continue losing weight and keeping it off.

The Bariatric diet is similar to the Paleo diet in some ways. Eat your proteins first, followed by the complex carbs from your fruits, vegetables, and legumes. You should be consuming 60 to 80 grams of protein a day, and initially 500 to 800 calories a day. As your body heals, you may be able to tolerate more. Usually, when your calorie intake consistently exceeds 1,000 to 1,200 calories for women and 1,400 to 1,600 for men, weight loss normally stalls. So, for as long as you can possibly can, maintain less than 1,000 calorie consumption daily.

The number of calories you need to maintain your weight depends on how much physical activity you do each day.

Eat three meals a day and one or two snacks. Keep a regular schedule with meals, always eating at the same times throughout the day, if possible. Do not go more than 5 waking hours without eating. As much as possible, plan and prepare your meals throughout the day to make it easier to eat healthy.

You may have caffeine in small quantities. Fried foods, fibrous vegetables, such as broccoli, and whole dairy products are off limits initially, but over time may be added in small portions. The same goes for candy, pastas, nuts, breads, and seeds. A big portion of the diet at this time should be mainly healthy fats, complex carbohydrates, and lean protein. Eliminate food with added sugar and processed food from their diet. Food should be chewed thoroughly and eaten slowly. You need to listen to the cues your body gives you and stop eating when no longer hungry.

Be mindful when you eat and do not be distracted–don't watch TV, work, drive, or play on your phone while eating; you may end up overeating without noticing. Like in the other phases, take your time when you eat. Each meal should be at least 20 minutes long, but not more than 30 minutes.

Keep your fluid intake at 48 to 64 ounces per day. Similar to the previous phases, avoid carbonated, high calorie, and caffeinated drinks. Do not use straws when drinking. You may have one cup of coffee or tea each day. While you may have caffeine now, decaf is preferred. Do not use high fat creamers or added sugar.

Continue keeping track of your food, fluids, and exercise in your food journal. Your food journal helps keep you on track and keeps records of food that your body tolerates. Aside from these, your food journal:

- Lets you know if you're meeting your nutritional needs.
- Helps you determine how each type of food can affect your fullness, energy levels, and moods.
- Shows you your emotional triggers that may turn you to eating for comfort.
- Keeps you accountable for your actions.
- Helps you create meal plans.
- Help you realize and celebrate your milestones.

Continue with your vitamins and supplements. You may now switch to tablets.

Continue with exercising at 30 to 45 minutes per session, 5 to 7 days out of the week. You may now add strength training to your routine, working up to 90 minutes of strength training per week. Strength training helps you build muscle mass, which, in turn, helps you burn more calories. Also add in balance training and stretching to maximize joint strength. Stretching helps prevent injuries and keeps you flexible,

With your surgery, there are some changes that you will be doing for a <u>lifetime</u>, such as:

- Taking certain vitamins and supplements. No gummy vitamins or supplements.
- No carbonated beverages allowed.

- Separating your meals from your fluid intake. Eating and drinking in one meal may cause dumping. In some people, drinking fluids while eating prevents them from listening to their fullness cues. In others, it causes them to be full too quickly and prevents them from getting enough nutrients. Some experience pain and nausea when eating and drinking at the same meal.

Dumping Syndrome

Dumping syndrome happens when food and fluids are rapidly emptied into the small intestine. This happens when you eat food that is too high in fat or sugar or if you eat too fast or too much.

Symptoms of dumping syndrome include:

- A strong desire to lie down
- Diarrhea
- Palpitations
- Nausea
- Lightheadedness
- Vomiting
- Flushing
- Pain
- Headache
- Abdominal cramps
- Sweating
- Bloating
- Epigastric fullness

To avoid dumping syndrome, avoid food that has too much sugar or food that has a high fat content. Separate your food intake with your fluid intake by one hour. When consuming fluids, do not use a straw, and do not drink carbonated beverages. Straws and carbonated beverages introduce air into your system and cause gas pains.

Avoid full fat dairy products. Opt for the low fat variety instead. Avoid pizza, ice cream, crackers, cookies, bread, juices, pasta, and rice. Avoid high fat meat items such as pepperoni, hot dogs, bacon, burgers, or pork sausages.

Chapter 1: The Liquid Diet and Sample Meal Plans

This section features sample meal plans for each phase of recovery after your surgery. Throughout each phase, emphasis on protein intake is given. Protein intake is so important that you have to track your consumption <u>daily</u> to make sure you meet your daily needs! Why is protein so important after your surgery?

Protein is the most important nutrient for those who have undergone bariatric surgery. It is part of each cell in your body. Every day, protein in your cells is being broken down and replaced. Your body is unable to store protein, so it is necessary to replenish the protein in your body through your diet. If you do not get enough protein, your body breaks down muscles to make up for the nutritional deficiency.

After gastric sleeve surgery, losing muscle is inevitable because of low calorie intake, but muscle loss can be minimized by making sure you have enough protein in your diet.

What does protein do for your body? Protein helps with wound healing. It builds and repairs tissues, such as those in your major organs, muscles, and skin.

Protein helps orchestrate a healthier weight loss by allowing your body to burn the fat in your body instead of muscle. When there is a drastic deficiency in calorie intake, your body protects itself by going into starvation mode and preserving its fat storage. It instead uses lean muscle mass for energy before it uses the fat stored in your body. If you meet your daily protein needs, you preserve your muscles from being used as energy, forcing your body to use your fat stores. This method is called protein sparing.

As mentioned earlier, protein helps build muscles in your body. The more muscles you have, the higher your metabolism is, so more calories are burned throughout the day, even when you're not being active.

Eating protein fills you up faster and longer. While during the first few weeks after your surgery, you won't be hungry much, your appetite will return eventually. If you make a habit of filling up on protein first, you resist grazing, which can lead to weight gain.

Protein builds your nails, skin, and hair, keeping them healthy. It also aids in creating immune system antibodies, enzymes, and hormones, helping your whole body function properly.

The amount of protein you need daily depends on your overall health, age, sex, how active you are, and the amount of lean muscle mass in the body. Right after surgery, since your stomach is smaller and you need to adjust to your new diet, your daily protein needs are 40 to 60 grams each day. Once you're moved on to solid food, your protein needs increase to 60 to 80 grams daily.

Since your digestive system can't handle solid food until a couple of months after surgery, protein shakes and powders are very important to make sure your body meets its daily protein needs, and to minimize lean muscle mass loss, and help wound healing. Even when you can start incorporating solid forms of protein in your diet, drinking protein shakes and adding protein powder in your diet is a convenient, fast, and easy way to meet your daily protein needs. Bear in mind, however, that while drinking your protein may be fast and convenient, it will not be as filling as solid forms of protein.

Since your body can only absorb a maximum of 30 grams at one time, it is important to spread out your protein intake throughout the day through your meals and snacks. Always make it a point to eat your protein first in every meal, in case you get full quickly.

Post-surgery, there are some patients who find digesting protein from animal meat such as chicken breast, beef, lamb, and pork, difficult. Many find chicken thighs tolerable to their healing stomach. If you are one of these people, wait around three months before you start including these types of protein into your diet.

Go for lean meats and avoid those high in fat. Also, choose the tender cuts of meat, to make digestion easier.

Amino acids build proteins. To keep our bodies at peak health, we need nine essential amino acids. These amino acids cannot be produced by our bodies, therefore, we need to get them through diet. We get these amino acids through animal protein such as dairy, beef, eggs, poultry, fish, seafood, and pork.

While some vegetables also contain protein, they are considered incomplete proteins since they don't contain all nine amino acids your body needs. Some examples of plant-based proteins are:

- Vegetables
- Beans
- Grains and rice
- Split peas and lentils

- Seeds and nuts

If you are a vegan, in order to get all nine of the needed amino acids, you should combine your plant-based proteins, such as eating beans with rice, or whole wheat bread with peanut butter. This is not the optimum way to get your protein, however, since most plant-based proteins are also high in calories, carbohydrates, or fat, and lower in protein content compared to animal proteins.

It is possible to be vegan after gastric sleeve surgery, but your diet will be higher in calories since you will need to combine several plant-based proteins to get the sufficient amino acids in your diet.

One plant-based protein, however, contains all the amino acids your body needs, and that is soy. Soy comes in various forms such as soybeans, tempeh, and tofu. In one cup of soybeans, you get 22 grams of protein and 250 calories. It also contains phytochemicals, vitamins and minerals, fiber, calcium, and iron. Studies show regular consumption of soy helps improve health issues such as (*Bariatric Nutrition and Lifestyle Plan*, 2017):

- Menopausal symptoms such insomnia, night sweats, and hot flashes
- Heart disease
- Certain cancers
- High blood pressure
- Osteoporosis

Soy can be consumed in many forms—as whole beans or edamame—or processed as soy milk, tofu, miso, tempeh, soy yogurt, and other soy-based products.

Soy as tofu also comes in various forms:

- Silken tofu: a creamy type of tofu and is used in dishes where you need to blend the tofu.
- Soft tofu: also used in dishes where you need to blend the tofu.
- Firm: Denser and has more calcium, fats, and protein than the other two. Firm tofu is often used in soups, cubed and stir-fried, barbecued, grilled, baked, scrambled, smoked, and pickled.

A second-best option are lupini beans. These are native to Italy and are part of the legume family. They are yellow, large, round, flat seeds. In Latin American and the Mediterranean Basin, these are usually pickled and eaten as a snack food. They are sold in jars and brined like olives and pickles. You can eat the thick outer skin, as it contains insoluble bran fiber.

Although it's not a complete source of the needed amino acids, it has most of them. Lupini beans are composed of 21% fat, 34% carbs, and 45% protein. One cup of lupini beans contain 26 grams of protein and 200 calories. It is high in antioxidants and amino acids such as arginine. It provides your body with lots of minerals and vitamins, especially B complex. It is gluten free, and low in cholesterol and fat. It also promotes the growth of good bacteria in your gut (*Bariatric Nutrition and Lifestyle Plan*, 2017).

It is a great snack food for diabetics, as it has a low glycemic index. For someone who has undergone gastric sleeve surgery, it is easy to digest.

Many people think you can get sufficient protein from seeds, nuts, and legumes. Unfortunately, this is not the case. While they do have protein, seeds, nuts, and legumes are high in carbohydrates and fat, and do not contain all the amino acids you need. These should not be considered as your main source of protein.

Legumes include lentils, peas, and beans. They are a great source of complex carbs (70%), protein (27%), essential vitamins, minerals, and fiber. One cup of legumes contains 240 calories and 15 grams of protein. You can add protein powder when eating legumes to meet your protein needs for the day.

Nuts and seeds provide you with phytochemicals, fiber, and vitamins and minerals. They are a great source of heart-healthy fat, plant protein, and calories. Nuts and seeds are composed of 72% fat, 15% carbs, and 13% protein. One cup of nuts or seeds contains 25 grams of protein and 800 calories. Nuts and seeds are good for your heart, however, eat them in moderation since they are high in calories.

Dairy is a great source of protein! Make sure, however, that you get the nonfat or low fat kinds.

Cheese has vitamin B12, calcium, vitamin A, phosphorus, and zinc. It is composed of 70% fat, 6% carbs, and 23% protein. On average, an ounce of cheese has 6 grams of saturated fat, 7 grams of protein, and 100 calories. The downside is that cheese is very high in saturated fat, so minimize it in your diet.

Assessing where to get your protein from may be challenging in the beginning. Look for sources that are high in protein and low in calories—for every 100 calories, there should be at least 10 grams of protein.

If you are getting hungry soon after eating a meal, it may be due to:

- Too much time has passed between meals
- The carbs you ate have been burned
- You didn't eat a sufficient enough amount of protein and complex carbs
- The protein you had was a soft food or in liquid form

Week 1: Clear Liquid Diet

During the first week, you will be following the same liquid diet that you were on days prior to surgery. This is to make sure that you don't suffer from any postoperative complications such as dehydration, bowel obstruction, constipation, gastric leakage, or diarrhea.

This week, drink lots of clear liquids. It is recommended that you have an intake of 48 to 64 ounces of fluids per day. Should you still feel dehydrated, discuss with your doctor on adding beverages with electrolytes, like sugar-free Gatorade.

It is important to not drink <u>anything</u> with sugar during this week! Sugar may cause dumping syndrome, an issue that occurs when too much sugar enters the small intestine too quickly. When this happens, vomiting, nausea, diarrhea, and fatigue occurs. Also, sugar is full of empty calories, something that should be minimized as part of the change in lifestyle post-surgery.

Beverages with caffeine such as coffee and tea should also be avoided, as these may cause dehydration and acid reflux.

No carbonated beverages may be consumed during this time as these types of beverages cause bloating and gas.

Here are some ideas of what beverages you can consume during this time:

- Diluted or light juices with artificial sweeteners. Limit your intake to this type of beverage to just 2 cups a day, because juices are heavy in calories.
  - Cranberry
  - Grape
  - Apple
- Clear broths made from
  - Chicken
  - Beef
  - Vegetable
  - Seafood
- Other
  - Water
  - Ice chips
  - Sugar free sports drinks
  - Decaffeinated tea

- Decaffeinated coffee
- Sugar-free non-carbonated flavored waters
- Sugar-free popsicles or frozen juice bars
- Sugar-free gelatin

Week 2: Liquid Diet

The second week post-op will allow you to have a full liquid diet. Keeping to this liquid diet will allow your stomach to heal, without stretching it.

Keep your fluid intake at 48 to 64 ounces each day. During this week, you may experience more hunger compared to the first week after your operation. Bear in mind, however, that your system still cannot handle solid food at this time. No carbonated beverages or caffeine is allowed during this week either. Avoid sugar and fat as well.

Try to get at least 40 grams of protein each day, more if you can tolerate it. Protein helps our body heal faster. Keep your calories at around 300 to 400 per day, at 4 to 6 meals a day. Keep your meals at 2 to 4 ounces each.

Take at least 20 minutes to eat, but no more than 30 minutes, and be mindful of each sip, assessing whether you are already full or with each one. <u>Do not feel the need to finish what is given to you if you are already full</u>.

Sip your fluids—no gulping. Separate your clear liquids from your full liquid meals. At this stage, you are allowed to drink clear liquids right after your full liquid meals.

Don't forget to log your food consumption in your food journal.

Here is a sample 7-day menu for week 2. Each beverage is a one cup serving, wherein one cup is equal to 8 fluid ounces.

DAY 1	DAY 2	DAY 3	DAY 4	DAY 5	DAY 6	DAY 7
Ensure Light	Sugar Free Vanilla Mint Smoothie	Basil and Blueberries Flavored Water	Instant Breakfast Drink	Mango Vanilla Smoothie	Cucumber and Mint Flavored Water	Unsweetened Milk
Water	Water	Water	Water	Water	Water	Water
Cherry Mango Smoothie	Watermelon Flavored Water	Non-fat plain Greek yogurt	Peach smoothie	Strawberries and sugar-free lemonade flavored water	Thinned cream of wheat	Strawberry banana smoothie
Water	Water	Water	Water	Water	Water	Water

Sugar-free cheesecake pudding	Thinned oatmeal	Sugar-free raspberry sorbet	Classic hummus	Lime sherbet freeze	Cottage cheese fluff	Fluffy jello
Water	Water	Water	Water	Water	Water	Water
Plain sugar-free yogurt	Slurpee	Pudding	Sherbet	Jello	Sugar-free ice cream	Apple sauce
Water	Water	Water	Water	Water	Water	Water

If any of the food you're eating feels like it's getting stuck, do not drink to try to push it down! Doing so might cause you to regurgitate the food or cause more discomfort. Walk around instead.

Spread out your protein intake into smaller servings, but more frequent meals, rather than consuming it all in one meal. You may pre-make your protein drinks and store them in the refrigerator and drink at your convenience. Set a timer to remind you when to eat and drink. Remember to make your meal last to at least 20 minutes to ensure you don't eat too fast. Listen to your body; if you feel full, stop eating or drinking and do not feel like you need to finish what was given to you.

Make sure you measure the protein you consume to ensure you are eating a sufficient amount every day. Same thing with your fluid intake; make sure it is measured to avoid dehydration. If you are getting enough fluids, your urine should be light yellow in color.

Some patients find water has a metallic taste to it. If you are one of them, just add some flavoring to your water to remedy this problem. Some also experience sensitivity to beverages that are hot or cold. Find what works best for you by experimenting.

Week 3: Pureed Food

During this week, you may progress onto pureed foods. Transitioning from liquid to pureed food before moving on to soft food allows your digestive system to adjust. Your calorie intake should be around 300 to 500 calories a day at three meals with one or two snacks. Protein intake should be from animal meat and at least 40 grams each day, or more if you can tolerate it. However, listen to your body. Sometimes two or three bites is enough in the beginning. As time goes on, increase the quantity if you can tolerate it.

Food should still be low-fat and sugar-free, as well as non-fibrous. Even though your food is already pureed, it is important to chew the food well. Start making it a habit to chew your food at least 25 times, and eat slowly. Make sure to breathe after each bite. Your meals should take at least 20 minutes long. Eat your food in dime-sized bites and sip your fluids slowly, no gulping.

You can start consuming fruits and vegetables during this phase. Avoid vegetables that are too fibrous or stringy, and make sure they are always cooked. Do not eat fruit with its skin on or that have any seeds that could potentially get stuck.

Never go more than 5 waking hours without eating. Even when you're not hungry, just take a few bites of food to maintain your eating schedule.

Continue with avoiding caffeine and food that is chunky. To avoid heartburn, the food should have little to no seasoning. Avoid eating hard cheeses at this phase. Also don't eat candy, pasta, ice cream, rice, pastries, bread, or crackers.

Make sure you drink 48 to 64 ounces of fluid daily. Protein shakes do not count towards your fluid intake. If you feel constipated, increase your fluid intake and try walking.

Following is a 7-day menu for week 3. All food should be pureed to the consistency of applesauce—no chunks. Puree meat with milk, broth, or water until the consistency of applesauce is achieved. Should you not like the taste of pureed meat, you may substitute it for eggs or protein shakes. Bear in mind that your stomach is still in the process of healing, and eating solid food may cause dumping syndrome or pain.

You may add protein powder to your food when you puree it to boost the protein content. You may add herbs and spices to enhance the flavor of your pureed food.

Take it easy on your system. Start off slow, with ¼ to ⅓ cup of food. Listen to your body for fullness cues. And if something doesn't feel right when you're eating, stop.

Introduce new food one at a time so you can make a note of how your body reacts to it. If you experience any gas, bloating, or nausea when eating new food, your body may not be ready for it at this time. Wait a few more days before trying it again.

Continue logging your food and fluid intake and physical activity in your food journal.

The most important change here is to separate your food intake from your fluid intake. Do not drink anything 15 minutes before you're about to eat, and wait an hour after eating before you drink anything.

	DAY 1	DAY 2	DAY 3	DAY 4	DAY 5	DAY 6	DAY 7
Drink 1	Water	Water	Water	Water	Water	Water	Water
Breakfast	Scrambled egg Peach with no skin	Apple avocado baby food	Silken tofu	Avocado spread	Cauliflower puree	Tomato soup and cottage cheese	Butternut squash baby food
Drink 2	Blackberry flavored water	Pineapple coconut flavored	Fruit punch flavored	Blue & black berry flavored	Orange mango flavored	Pomegranate cranberry flavor	Pear flavored red water

			water	d water	water	water	ed water	
Drink3	Water	Water	Water	Water	Water	Water	Water
Lunch	Pureed cooked white fish	Cream of chicken soup	Pumpkin mousse	Soft boiled egg	Apple sauce	Bean spread	Pureed chicken thigh with sweet potatoes
Drink4	Diluted Tomato juice	Diluted Pomegranate juice	Green tea	Diluted Cranberry juice	Diluted Acai berry juice	Diluted Blackberry juice	Diluted Strawberry juice
Drink5	Water	Water	Water	Water	Water	Water	Water
Snack	Chocolate protein shake	Apple cherry baby food	Banana baby food	Lemon mousse	Apple baby food	Cottage cheese	Avocado mousse

Drink 6	Peppermint flavored water	Diluted Blueberry juice	Rose flavored water	Strawberry watermelon flavored water	Coconut water	Lavender flavored water	Passion fruit flavored water
Drink 7	Water	Water	Water	Water	Water	Water	Water
Dinner	Cream of mushroom soup	Carrot baby food	Hummus	Plain Greek yogurt	Cream of potato soup	Skim milk with protein powder	Pureed beef
Drink 8	Water	Water	Water	Water	Water	Water	Water

If any of the food you're eating feels like it's getting stuck, do not drink to try to push it down. Doing so might cause you to regurgitate the food or cause more discomfort. Walk around instead.

Weeks 4 to 5: Soft Food

Weeks 4 and 5 post-surgery marks the introduction of soft food into your diet. Your food no longer needs to be pureed, but stick to food that is moist and tender. Since the food is now more solid, you have to make an effort to really chew your food thoroughly.

Trim any visible fat off the meat you're eating. Avoid the skin from chicken and other poultry, as these are high in fat. Meat should be moist and soft enough to swallow without feeling like it "sticks." Keep to meats that are boiled and marinated, and for chicken, stick to dark meat, as it is more tender. Avoid meat that is fibrous, like steak, chicken breast, or dry turkey.

When cooking meat, do not grill or microwave, as these dry out the meat. Do not fry the meat. Frying adds unnecessary calories to your food, makes the food hard to digest, and may cause you to have dumping syndrome.

You may use a microwave to reheat meat, but add some chicken broth or water to add more juice to the meat, since meat stored in the refrigerator also has a tendency to dry out. Using a slow cooker is the best way to cook meat at this time, as it keeps it moist and tender. You may also steam, bake, or broil your meat.

Always cook your vegetables well. Make sure they are soft. Do not eat any fibrous vegetables such as pea pods, celery, corn, and cucumbers, which are hard to digest.

You may eat frozen and canned fruit, but make sure the canned fruit is packed in its own juice and not in syrup. Drain the fruit before consuming.

While you may eat grapefruit, tangerines, and oranges, do not eat the membranes (the white parts), as these are hard to digest. Also avoid eating the core, seeds, and skins of fruits such as tomatoes, apples, berries, and grapes.

You may eat soft cheeses during this phase.

Fat, sugar, and high carb foods should still be avoided, and keep your diet to soft food. Continue to avoid food that's hard to digest, such as nuts, fruits or vegetables high in fiber, or steak. Here is a sample 7-day menu for week 4. You may find recipes for some of the dishes in the sample menu below in this book.

	DAY 1	DAY 2	DAY 3	DAY 4	DAY 5	DAY 6	DAY 7
Breakfast	Scrambled eggs with pureed kale and cheese	Boiled sweet potato	Cottage cheese and mashed melon	Cooked cereal	Low fat, sliced turkey breast	Cooked beans	Softened, unsweetened cereal in milk
Lunch	Chickpea salad	Egg drop soup	Steamed grouper	Texas hash	Chopped turkey breast	Lemon garlic tilapia	Potato soup
Snack	Creamy garlic herb mashed	Goat cheese	Banana	Low fat ham and mozzarella	Hard boiled egg	Baked potato	Canned peaches

				cheese			
	potatoes						
Dinner	Dairy-free cheesy zucchini rice	Baked chicken	Split pea and ham soup	Sautéed ground beef with chayote	Classic meat loaf	Steamed shrimp	Parmesan herb crusted baked salmon

Make sure to stop drinking fluids 15 minutes before eating a meal or snack, and wait an hour after eating before drinking anything.

If any of the food you're eating feels like it's getting stuck, do not drink to try to push it down. Doing so might cause you to regurgitate the food or cause more discomfort. Walk around instead.

Introduce new food to your digestive system one at a time, so you can assess the effect it has on your system and see if it is well-tolerated. It is recommended to try new food when you're at home on the weekends, just in case your system doesn't tolerate the new food well.

During the beginning of this phase, you might not be able to eat the required amount of protein, so you may supplement your diet with protein shakes and powders.

Week 6 Onwards: Solid Food

Week 6 is when you start eating solid food. Keep your diet to nutrient-dense vegetables and lean protein. It is important to slowly introduce the different foods to your body so you can take note if there is an adverse reaction. Avoid soda, processed food, and food with added sugars. You may eat everything else unless your body has a reaction to it.

Always keep yourself hydrated. Eat small meals and minimize snacking. Here is a sample 7-day menu for week 6. The dishes in the sample menu below can be found in this book.

	DAY 1	DAY 2	DAY 3	DAY 4	DAY 5	DAY 6	DAY 7
Breakfast	Pumpkin bread	Blueberry and cottage cheese pancakes	Cinnamon swirl loaf	Denver omelette	Vegan vanilla buttermilk pancakes	Spanish tortilla with ham	Lemon and poppy seed loaf
Lunch	Cheesy chicken enchilada soup	Pulled pork	Avocado tuna salad sandwich	Roasted garlic potato soup	Cream of chicken soup	Asian pork tenderloin	Apple and tuna sandwich
Snack	Chee	Apple	Quin	Vanill	Apple	Sticky	Blue

k	sy potato and turkey pancakes	carrot bread	oa fruit salad with honey lemon dressing	a mug cake	zucchini bread	lemon cake	berry sour cream cake
Dinner	Couscous chicken soup	Shepherd's pie	Pan fried trout	Vegetarian fried rice	Chicken with peanut apple sauce	Pork and black bean stew	Shrimp ceviche

Like in the previous phases, eat your food and drink your beverages separately. You may drink right up to when you're about to eat, but not during mealtime. You also need to wait one hour after eating before you can start drinking.

You may now eat vegetables and fruits that are high in fiber.

Chapter 2: Soft Food Recipes

Aside from the recipes listed in this chapter, you may also eat the following foods while on a soft food diet. Remember the foods from earlier that you need to avoid or limit (caffeine, excess sugar, fatty foods).

Dairy: Keep away from whole dairy products, but you can eat:

- Cheeses that are sliced thinly or melted
- Yogurt
- Ricotta or cottage cheese
- Ice cream
- Milk and milkshakes

Grains: Keep away from high fiber grains, but you can eat:

- Soft or moist cereals
- Saltine crackers in soup
- Rice

Proteins:

- Baked beans
- Eggs—hard or soft boiled, scrambled, poached
- Tofu
- Chopped or ground poultry and fish
- Small pieces of meat in broth or soup

Fruits and vegetables: Keep away from fruits and vegetables that are high in fiber, but you can eat:

- Applesauce
- Soft, cooked vegetables
- Drained canned fruit
- Soft fruit eaten with no skin (e.g. watermelon, peaches, bananas)
- Cooked or baked fruits

Avoid foods that are sticky, tough, hard, or crunchy while at this stage. Do not eat spicy food either, as this may cause bloating and upset your stomach.

Avoid the following foods while on a soft food diet:

Proteins:

- Peanut butter (both crunchy and creamy variants)
- Steak
- Hot dogs
- Beef jerky
- Sausages
- Bacon

Starches:

- Popcorn
- Hard cereal, crackers, toast
- Bread
- Anything with seeds, nuts, or dried fruits
- Hard chips
- Uncooked potatoes

Fruits:

- Skin of fruit
- Hard fruits, like apples or pears
- Stringy fruits, like mango or pineapple

Vegetables

- Hard, raw, or vegetables that are not mashed
- Corn on the cob
- Peas

Soft Food Preparation

When eating the foods mentioned above, it needs to be prepped so the food doesn't have to be chewed up as much. Here are some ways to go about this:

- Mash the food.
- Cut the food into tiny pieces
- Puree or grind the food.
- Moisten the food with sauce, gravy, or broth.

Poultry Dishes

Scrambled Eggs With Pureed Kale and Cheese

The recipe calls for nutrient-packed kale. Should you not find any kale available, you may substitute with spinach, which is very nutritious as well.

Cheese is used in this dish. You can use any of your favorite cheese that melts easily. This also uses Italian seasoning, but this will work well with any seasoning of your choice.

Time: 15 minutes

Serving Size: 2

Prep Time: 10 minutes

Cook Time: 5 minutes

Ingredients:

- 1 tbsp extra virgin olive oil
- ¼ cup finely chopped onion
- 1 cup fresh kale, pureed
- 4 medium eggs, beaten
- ½ tsp Italian seasoning

- ½ cup shredded low-fat cheese (pick a cheese that melts easily, such as mozzarella, cheddar, swiss, provolone, or gruyere)
- Salt and pepper

Directions:

1. Heat the oil in a pan over medium heat.
2. Once the oil is hot, sauté the onions for one minute.
3. Add the pureed kale and cook with the onions for a few minutes.
4. Lower to medium heat then add the beaten eggs. Stir the eggs until they begin to solidify.
5. Add the italian seasoning and shredded cheese. Continue cooking until the cheese is melted and the eggs are cooked to desired doneness.
6. Season with salt and pepper to taste.

Egg Drop Soup

If you're in a rush and need something that can be prepared quickly, but also bel delicious and nutritious, this soup is perfect! It just takes 15 minutes to prep and cook, and you probably already have the ingredients on hand. Easy to prepare and relatively inexpensive, this soup is also perfect to eat during a rainy day.

Time: 15 minutes

Serving Size: 4

Prep Time: 5 minutes

Cook Time: 10 minutes

Ingredients:

- 1 tbsp soy sauce
- 1 tsp ground ginger
- 32 ounces chicken broth
- 2 eggs, beaten
- 2 green onions, chopped
- Salt and pepper

Directions:

1. Combine soy sauce, ginger, and chicken broth in a saucepan and let it simmer.
2. Slowly pour in the eggs while stirring the soup.
3. Add the green onions, salt, and pepper.

(Optional)

4. If you want a thicker broth, you may mix a tablespoon of cornstarch to two tablespoons of chicken broth, then slowly add to the simmering soup.

Pork and Beef Dishes

Split Pea and Ham Soup

This soup uses the bone from a ham to add to the flavor. It also uses split peas, which are very nutritious and full of soluble fiber that helps keep your blood sugar stable and lower your cholesterol levels. Split peas are also very filling, and can make you feel full faster and longer. This is a nutritious, low-fat soup you can indulge in.

Split peas, much like dried beans, require a long cooking time. To speed things up a bit, you may soak the peas in water overnight to start the softening process.

You can make a big batch of this soup and store it in the freezer, as it freezes very well. After cooking the soup, let it cool, the place in freezer containers and store in the freezer. If you want to eat the soup for lunch or dinner, let it thaw overnight in the refrigerator. Add a little chicken broth or water should the soup be too thick for your liking, then heat over the stove in a pot, or in a bowl in the microwave for a few minutes.

Time: 8 hours and 10 minutes

Serving Size: 8

Prep Time: 10 minutes

Cook Time: 8 hours

Ingredients:

- 6 cups low-sodium chicken broth + more if needed

- 16 ounce bag green split peas, rinsed and drained
- 1 ham bone, with about 1 pound of meat
- 2 carrots, peeled and finely chopped
- 2 celery stalks, finely chopped
- 1 bay leaf
- ½ cup yellow or white onion, finely chopped
- 1 tbsp fresh thyme, finely chopped
- 1 tbsp garlic, minced
- ⅓ cup fresh Italian flat leaf parsley, finely chopped
- Salt and black pepper to taste

Directions:

1. In the slow cooker, layer the ingredients in this order:

o Split peas

o Carrots

o Celery

o Onion

o Garlic

o Parsley

o Thyme

o Bay leaf

o Salt and pepper

o Ham bone

2. Add enough chicken broth to cover the ingredients in the slow cooker. Cover.

3. Cook for 8 to 10 hours on low, stirring occasionally.

4. Once the peas are soft, remove the ham bone and bay leaf from the slow cooker.

5. Remove the meat off the bone. Finely chop the ham and place back in the slow cooker.

6. Mash the peas and stir. If needed, you may add more broth until you reach the desired consistency of the soup.

7. Add salt and pepper to taste.

Classic Meatloaf

Chopping all the ingredients may take some time, so it's best to pull out the vegetable chopper or food processor if you're in a hurry. Make sure the vegetables are chopped as small as possible, so the meat loaf holds together well.

You may substitute ground beef with ground turkey.

When baking the meatloaf, make sure that it is baking at a low heat so that the outside of the meat loaf doesn't dry out and burn before the inside cooks sufficiently. To know if the meatloaf is done, the center temperature should be at least 155°F.

Time: 1 hour 30 minutes

Serving Size: 4

Prep Time: 20 minutes

Cook Time: 1 hour 10 minutes

Ingredients:

- 2 tbsp unsalted butter
- 1 tbsp garlic, minced
- 1 cup onion, finely chopped
- ½ cup green onion, finely chopped
- 1 celery stalk, finely chopped
- 1 carrot, finely chopped
- Salt and pepper
- ⅔ cup ketchup, divided into 2 equal parts

- 2 tsp Worcestershire sauce
- 1/3 cup fresh parsley leaves, minced
- 1 cup breadcrumbs
- 2 ¼ pounds of ground beef
- 2 large eggs, beaten

Directions:

1. Place the rack in the middle of the oven, and preheat your oven to 350°F.
2. Place the butter in a pan and melt over medium heat. Once the butter has melted, add the garlic, onions, green onions, celery, and carrots to the pan. Cook for 5 minutes, stirring occasionally.
3. Cover the pan and let it cook until the carrots are soft, around 5 more minutes. Stir occasionally.
4. Season the vegetables with salt and pepper. Add the first half of the ketchup and the Worcestershire sauce. Cook for 1 minute, then set aside to cool.
5. In a large bowl, mix the parsley, cooked vegetables, breadcrumbs, ground beef, and eggs with your hands until all the ingredients are evenly combined.
6. Press the meat mixture in a loaf pan (5x9 inch or 4x8 inch pan) to make it compact. Cover the top of the meat mixture with the remaining ketchup.
7. Bake at 350°F until the meat thermometer reads 155°F when inserted in the center. This should take about an hour.

8. Remove the meatloaf from the oven and let it cool for 10 minutes. Then lift the meatloaf out of the pan with a metal spatula.

9. Cut into thick slices when serving.

Texas Hash

This dish is made with tomatoes, ground beef, rice, and bell peppers, all cooked in just one skillet. Not only is the dish easy to make, clean up is also a breeze since it is a one-pot dish! If you're a cheese lover like me, you may add some low fat grated cheese on top to add to the flavor and make the dish creamier.

This is a filling, hearty, and mouthwatering dish that will surely be one of your favorites.

Time: 30 minutes

Serving Size: 4

Prep Time: 5 minutes

Cook Time: 25 minutes

Ingredients:

- 2 tbsp olive oil
- 1 pound ground beef
- 1 cup diced onion
- 1 tbsp garlic, minced
- 2 tsp salt
- ¼ tsp ground pepper
- 1 cup green bell pepper, diced
- ½ tsp dry mustard
- ½ cup uncooked white rice

- 2 tbsp tomato paste
- 1 tsp Worcestershire sauce
- 1 cup water
- 1 can (14.5 ounces) diced tomatoes with juice
- 1 cup cheddar cheese, shredded

Directions:

1. Heat oil over medium high heat in a pan that has a tight fitting cover.
2. Sauté the beef until it is no longer pink. Make sure you break it up as it cooks.
3. Drain the beef of the excess oil and add the onions. Sauté until fragrant, about two or three minutes.
4. Add the garlic and sauté for a minute, then add the salt, pepper, bell pepper, and dry mustard, combine well.
5. Add the rice and allow it to absorb the liquid in the pan for a couple of minutes.
6. Pour in the tomato paste and cook for another minute.
7. Add the Worcestershire sauce, water, and canned tomatoes with the juice. Mix well, cover, and let it simmer for 20 minutes.
8. Fluff the rice. If it is still too wet, cook with the lid off for a few more minutes until you've reached desired consistency.
9. Add the cheese on top and cook for two or three more minutes to let the cheese melt a little.

Fish and Seafood Dishes

Parmesan Herb Crusted Baked Salmon

This is an easy and quick dish to prepare, but elegant enough that you can serve it at a dinner party. This salmon dish pairs well with a side of roasted vegetables and rice. You may also serve it with green beans and some mashed potatoes.

If you are not a fan of parsley, you may opt to use chopped cilantro instead.

Time: 17 minutes

Serving Size: 4

Prep Time: 2 minutes

Cook Time: 15 minutes

Ingredients:

- 1 2 pound whole salmon fillet
- ½ cup Parmesan cheese, chopped
- ¼ cup parsley, chopped
- 3 cloves garlic, finely minced

Directions:

1. Line your baking sheet with aluminum foil or parchment paper so clean up will be easier after cooking.
2. Preheat the oven to 425°F.

3. Mix the parmesan cheese, parsley, and garlic together to make a paste.
4. Put the salmon filet skin side down on the baking sheet then cover it with a sheet of parchment paper, then place in the oven and bake for 10 minutes.
5. Take the salmon out of the oven and remove the parchment paper. Top the salmon with the parmesan cheese paste and place back in the oven to cook for another 5 minutes, until the fish has reached an internal temperature of 135°F, the flesh flakes easily, and the cheese has melted and has lightly browned.
6. Let the fish rest for 5 minutes before serving.

Lemon Garlic Tilapia

This fish dish is quick to make and is cooked in just one pan, making clean up a breeze. Instead of tilapia, you may use sol, pollack, or flounder.

You can add a layer of fresh vegetables underneath while it's cooking in the oven to make the dish more nutritious. You can also add a little bit of dill to this to make it more tangy.

This dish goes well with some yellow rice, sweet potatoes, or pasta and a salad, some broccoli, or steamed bok choy.

Time: 40 minutes

Serving Size: 4

Prep Time: 10 minutes

Cook Time: 30 minutes

Ingredients:

- 4 tilapia fillets
- 3 tbsp lemon juice
- 1 tbsp butter, melted
- Salt and pepper
- 1 tsp dried parsley flakes
- 1 clove garlic, finely chopped

Directions:

1. Preheat your oven to 375°F.

2. Grease a baking dish and set aside.
3. Rinse the fish under running water and dry with paper towels.
4. Put the fish in the baking dish and pour the lemon juice and butter on the fillets. Sprinkle the salt, pepper, parsley, and garlic over the fish.
5. Place in the oven and bake until the fish gets flakey and turns white, which is around 30 minutes.

Vegetarian Dishes

Creamy Garlic Herb Mashed Potatoes

Potatoes are great to eat because they are so filling. For this dish, it is important that you don't include the skin. Your stomach is still healing and the skin on potatoes is too hard to digest.

The easiest way to mash all the ingredients together would be to take a hand mixer and whip the ingredients until smooth. The potatoes should be soft enough to mash this way after several hours in the slow cooker. Make sure there are no chunks in the mixture.

Time: 4 hours and 10 minutes

Serving Size: 6

Prep Time: 10 minutes

Cook Time: 4 hours

Ingredients:

- 2 lbs potatoes, washed
- ¼ cup almond milk
- 3 tbsp coconut oil mixed well with 1 tbsp water
- ½ tbsp lemon juice mixed well with ½ cup coconut milk
- 1 tsp pepper
- 1 tbsp garlic, finely chopped
- 2 tsp salt

- 1 tbsp minced fresh parsley or 2 tbsp flaked dried parsley
- ¼ tsp dried oregano
- ½ tsp fresh or dried basil

Directions:

1. Peel the potatoes, then chop into 2-inch pieces.
2. Grease your slow cooker with some coconut oil and place the potatoes in the slow cooker.
3. Cook for 5 to 6 hours on low or 2 to 3 hours on high.
4. Add the rest of the ingredients and combine well.
5. Mash the potatoes.

Dairy-Free Cheesy Zucchini Rice

This dish is so velvety, smooth, and creamy, I'm sure you'll be eating this even after the soft food phase. This goes well with many other dishes should you opt to use it as a side dish. For those who don't like vegetables much, the creaminess of the vegan cheese shines in this dish, so you won't notice the zucchini. Should you want less of the cheesiness and more of the vegetable flavor, scale back on the cheese and add more zucchini to the dish. Either way, this is a delicious way to get vegetables in your diet.

You can also substitute butternut squash instead of zucchini for this recipe.

Time: 30 minutes

Serving Size: 4

Prep Time: 10 minutes

Cook Time: 20 minutes

Ingredients:

- 2 cups vegetable broth
- 1 cup white rice
- Salt and pepper
- 2 cups zucchini, pureed
- ½ tsp garlic powder
- 1 cup shredded vegan cheddar cheese
- 1 to 2 tbsp almond milk

Directions:

1. Combine the broth and rice in a saucepan and bring to a boil.
2. Cover and lower the heat and let it simmer until the broth has been absorbed, around 15 to 20 minutes.
3. Turn off the heat and add in the salt and pepper, zucchini puree, garlic powder, and cheese.
4. If the sauce is too thick, you may add the milk to thin it out.

Chickpea Salad

This easy to prepare salad is sweet and savory. Try to make enough to have leftovers the next day, or prepare the salad the day before you plan on eating it, because once the ingredients and flavors start soaking in, it makes the salad a lot more flavorful.

To make the salad more nutritious, we added some kale. The salad has so much flavor, you won't even notice the bitterness of the kale. You can also chop up an apple and toss it in, or add some grapes with the salad to add some more crunch and sweetness to the dish.

Aside from eating this plain as a salad, you can also eat this as a wrap using a tortilla, collard, or lettuce. You can even spread it on toast and eat it as a sandwich!

For newbie vegans, this is a perfect transition from chicken salads. The texture and flavors are similar, but do not contain animal products.

You can use any kind of mustard for this recipe, or even substitute it with vegan mayonnaise. The amount of lemon juice to squeeze in there is really up to you, depending on how tart you want the salad to be.

Time: 30 minutes

Serving Size: 2

Prep Time: 25 minutes

Cook Time: 5 minutes

Ingredients:

- 1 can (15 oz) chickpeas, rinsed and drained
- 1 medium boiled carrot, shredded
- Juice from ½ of a lemon
- 2 celery stalks, cooked and finely chopped
- ½ tsp cooked and minced garlic
- ¼ cup red onion, cooked and finely chopped
- 2 to 3 tbsp dijon mustard
- ½ cup boiled kale, finely chopped
- 2 tbsp boiled cilantro, finely chopped
- Salt and pepper

Directions:
1. Mash the chickpeas until smooth in texture.
2. Add the rest of the ingredients.
3. Salt and pepper to taste.

Chapter 3: Solid Food Recipes– Breakfast

Vegetarian Dishes

Pumpkin Bread

This pumpkin bread is very moist. To keep yours as moist, you have to take the bread out of the pan once it's done baking and let it cool for 5 minutes. Then, wrap it in aluminum foil and let it cool further. Doing this keeps the moisture inside the bread. You should also use sugar, pumpkin puree, water, and oil to keep the bread moist. Adding the pumpkin spice and cinnamon gives the bread a heavenly, irresistible smell.

You may use either dark brown sugar, or light brown sugar. Not only will it change how brown the bread will be when done, but there is a slight difference in sweetness.

Time: 1 hour 15 minutes

Serving Size: 1 loaf

Prep Time: 15 minutes

Cook Time: 60 minutes

Ingredients:

- ½ tsp pumpkin spice
- ½ tsp cinnamon

- ½ cup granulated sugar
- ½ cup brown sugar
- ½ tsp salt
- 1 cup all-purpose flour
- ¾ tsp baking soda
- ½ tsp baking powder
- ⅓ cup water
- 1 large egg
- ⅓ cup oil
- ¾ cup pumpkin puree

Directions:

1. Preheat the oven to 350°F.
2. Combine the pumpkin spice, cinnamon, granulated sugar, brown sugar, salt, flour, baking soda, and baking powder in a bowl.
3. In a separate bowl, combine the water, egg, oil, and pumpkin puree, then add this mixture to the dry ingredients. Mix well.
4. Pour the batter into a greased 9x4-inch loaf pan and bake until a toothpick inserted in the middle of the loaf comes out clean, about 45 to 60 minutes.
5. Once the bread is done baking, take it out of the oven and let it sit in the pan for 5 minutes before taking it out and wrapping it in aluminum foil.

Vegan Vanilla Buttermilk Pancakes With Cinnamon

Time: 15 minutes

Serving Size: 4

Prep Time: 10 minutes

Cook Time: 5 minutes

Ingredients:

- ¼ tsp salt
- 2 cups all-purpose flour
- 1 tsp baking soda
- 3 tbsp white sugar
- 1 ½ tsp baking powder
- 4 tbsp lemon juice
- 2 cups almond milk
- 1 egg
- ½ tsp ground cinnamon
- 1 ½ tsp vanilla extract
- ¼ cup margarine, melted

Directions:

1. Whisk the salt, flour, baking soda, sugar, and baking powder in a bowl.

2. To make your vegan buttermilk, mix 4 tbsp lemon juice to 2 cups of almond milk. Let it stand for ten minutes to thicken.
3. In a separate bowl, mix the egg, vegan buttermilk, ground cinnamon, and vanilla. Add in the margarine.
4. Combine the wet and dry mixtures, mixing well. Don't overmix the batter, so your pancakes come out light and fluffy.
5. Preheat your pan over medium low heat. Grease the pan with a little bit of margarine.
6. Scoop ⅓ cup of batter onto the pan. Flip the pancake over once little bubbles start forming at the top, after about 3 minutes. Cook for another 2 minutes. Repeat until you run out of batter.

Cinnamon Swirl Loaf

This cinnamon swirl load is a delicious, moist, and soft cake that goes well with your coffee or tea. It is soft, fluffy, and easy to make.

This loaf freezes well. Slice the loaf into several pieces once it is baked and cooled completely, and store in the freezer.

Time: 1 hour

Serving Size: 1 loaf

Prep Time: 10 minutes

Cook Time: 50 minutes

Ingredients:

- 2 ½ tbsp lemon juice
- 1 ¼ cup almond milk + extra 2 tsp set aside
- ¼ cup canola oil
- 2 cups all-purpose flour
- 1 cup white sugar + extra ½ cup set aside
- 1 tsp vanilla extract
- 1 tsp baking powder
- ¼ cup silken tofu, pureed
- ½ tsp salt
- 1 tbsp cinnamon powder
- ¼ cup powdered sugar

Directions:

1. Preheat the oven to 350°F.
2. To make your vegan buttermilk, mix the lemon juice to 1 ¼ cups of almond milk. Let it stand for ten minutes and let it thicken.
3. Stir together the oil, flour, 1 cup sugar, vanilla, baking powder, tofu, salt, and vegan buttermilk.
4. In a separate bowl, combine the ½ cup sugar and cinnamon.
5. Grease a 9-inch loaf pan with some canola oil.
6. Pour half of your batter into a bread pan. Drizzle with half of the sugar-cinnamon powder. Pour in the other half of the batter, then sprinkle with the rest of the sugar-cinnamon powder. Using a knife, cut through the batter to swirl it.
7. Place the baking pan in the oven and bake until a toothpick inserted in the center of the load comes out clean, about 45 to 50 minutes.
8. Once done baking, take out of the oven and allow it to remain in the pan for 10 minutes before transferring the loaf to a wire rack to let it cool completely.
9. Mix the 2 tsp of almond milk and powdered sugar and drizzle over the loaf.

Lemon and Poppy Seed Loaf

Time: 1 hour 30 minutes

Serving Size: 1 loaf

Prep Time: 25 minutes

Cook Time: 1 hour 5 minutes

Ingredients:

- ¾ cup butter, softened
- 1 cup granulated sugar
- 1 tsp lemon extract
- 2 large eggs, beaten lightly
- 3 tbsp poppy seeds
- Zest from 1 lemon
- Juice from 1 lemon
- ¼ tsp salt
- 1 ¾ cups all-purpose flour
- 2 tsp baking powder
- ⅔ cup milk

Directions:

1. Preheat the oven to 325°F.
2. In a mixer, at a slow speed, combine the butter, sugar, and lemon extract together.
3. Pour in the eggs slowly.

4. Add the poppy seeds, lemon zest, and lemon juice.
5. Combine the salt, flour, and baking powder and mix well.
6. Add half of the flour and milk. Once blended well, add the rest of the flour and mix well.
7. Grease the baking pan and line with parchment paper.
8. Pour the batter into the baking pan and bake until a toothpick inserted into the center of the loaf comes out clean, about an hour to 1 hour and 5 minutes.
9. Once baked, take the pan out of the oven and let the loaf cool enough to transfer to a wire rack.

Pumpkin Pie Oatmeal

Time: 18 minutes

Serving Size: 1

Prep Time: 15 minutes

Cook Time: 3 minutes

Ingredients:

- ½ tsp salt
- ⅓ cup silken tofu
- 1 tsp lemon juice
- ¼ tbsp nutritional yeast
- ¼ tsp apple cider vinegar
- ⅓ cup firm tofu, crumbled
- 1 tsp sugar
- ⅓ cup oats
- Pinch of ground ginger
- Pinch of ground cloves
- ⅛ tsp cinnamon
- ½ cup canned pumpkin

Directions:

1. Prepare the vegan cottage cheese by pureeing salt, silken tofu, lemon juice, nutritional yeast, and apple cider vinegar in a blender.

2. Pour the silken tofu mixture into a bowl and combine with the crumbled firm tofu. Set this cottage cheese aside.
3. In a microwave safe bowl, mix the sugar, oats, ginger, cloves, cinnamon, and pumpkin.
4. Microwave for 90 seconds on high.
5. Add in the cottage cheese.
6. Microwave for another 60 seconds on high.
7. Let it cool down for a few minutes before consuming.

Non-Vegetarian Dishes

Blueberry and Cottage Cheese Pancakes

These pancakes are easy to make, light, sweet and buttery, and fluffy, bursting with blueberries with every bite. These are very filling and should keep you full all morning.

The cottage cheese in this recipe makes these pancakes healthier, as it increases the amount of protein in the dish. You can also add zest from one lemon and some chia seeds for added nutrients.

Instead of whole wheat flour, you can also use ground oatmeal.

Time: 20 minutes

Serving Size: 4

Prep Time: 10 minutes

Cook Time: 10 minutes

Ingredients:

- ¾ tsp salt
- 1 cup whole wheat flour
- 1 cup all-purpose flour
- ¾ tsp baking powder
- 3 tbsp brown sugar
- 1 ½ tsp baking soda

- 2 large eggs
- 2 tsp vanilla extract
- 1 cup cottage cheese
- 1 ½ cups whole milk
- 2 cups blueberries
- Butter

Directions:

1. Combine the salt, wheat flour and all-purpose flour, baking powder, brown sugar, and baking soda in a bowl.
2. In a separate bowl, beat the eggs and add the vanilla, cottage cheese, and milk. Mix well.
3. Add the egg mixture to the dry mixture and mix well.
4. Fold in the blueberries and combine evenly. Don't overmix the batter.
5. Grease the pan with a little butter.
6. Pour ⅓ cup of batter on a pan and flip over once small bubbles at the top form, at about the 3 minute mark. Then cook for another 1 to 2 minutes. Repeat until you run out of batter.

Denver Omelette

Combining the half and half with the eggs makes it light, fluffy, and buttery. The cheese and ham adds saltiness to the dish, while the onions and green pepper adds a slight sweetness to the dish.

This omelette can be customized with various ingredients and it will transform into a new dish each time. You can add chopped zucchini, different types of crumbled cheeses such as blue cheese or feta, chopped mushroom, and spinach.

You may top it with guacamole, pico de gallo, sour cream, or salsa. You can serve with biscuits and gravy, hash browns, fresh fruit, and sweet potato hash on the side.

Instead of using half and half, you can use milk or heavy whipping cream.

This dish freezes very well, so you can make a big batch, let it cool completely, then cover with plastic wrap or aluminum foil. This can be stored in the freezer for 3 to 6 months. You may thaw in the refrigerator overnight. Slice the omelette and reheat in the microwave for 30 seconds at a time until warmed sufficiently. You may also place the entire tray directly in the oven at 350°F for 10 minutes to reheat. You may also store it in the fridge, and it will be good for 3 to 4 days.

Time: 35 minutes

Serving Size: 6

Prep Time: 10 minutes

Cook Time: 25 minutes

Ingredients:

- 1 tbsp olive oil
- ½ cup green pepper
- ½ cup onion
- ½ cup half and half
- 8 eggs
- 1 cup cheddar cheese, shredded
- 1 cup cooked ham, chopped

Directions:

1. Preheat the oven to 400°F.
2. Heat olive oil over medium heat in a frying pan. Once the oil is hot, saute the green pepper and onion until it caramelizes a bit. Cooking the onion and green pepper reduces the moisture when it is baking with the eggs.
3. Mix the cream and eggs in a bowl. Add the green pepper, cheese, onion, and ham.
4. Put the mixture in a 9x9-inch baking pan and bake until golden brown, about 25 minutes.

Spanish Tortilla with Ham

Spanish tortillas can either be baked or fried. This recipe uses both methods—we saute some of the ingredients first, to caramelize and remove some of the moisture, before they are mixed in with the rest of the ingredients and baked. Baking the tortilla cooks it more evenly than if it was cooked in a pan, making it easier to flip over.

You can bake it in a rectangular baking pan, individual molds, or in a round baking pan.

While most would serve this as a breakfast or brunch dish, you may also serve it as an appetizer. If it is being served as a main dish, cut the tortilla in large slices, or bake in individual molds. If being served as an appetizer, slice the tortilla in square, bite sized pieces.

Sprinkle with shredded queso fresco and parsley when serving.

Time: 1 hour

Serving Size: 4

Prep Time: 15 minutes

Cook Time: 45 minutes

Ingredients:

- 3 tbsp olive oil
- 1 pound potatoes, peeled and sliced
- 3 garlic cloves, crushed
- 1 onion, sliced

- 12 ounces ham, sliced into thin strips
- Salt and pepper
- 8 eggs
- Queso fresco, crumbled
- Parsley, chopped

Directions:

1. Preheat the oven to 375°F.
2. Over medium heat, heat the olive oil in a pan. Cook the potatoes for 5 to 7 minutes, tossing occasionally.
3. Add the garlic and onions, stirring occasionally and cook for 10 minutes.
4. Mix in the ham with the other ingredients and cook until the potatoes are tender, for about 5 minutes. Add salt to taste.
5. Set aside and let the mixture cool for 5 minutes.
6. Beat the eggs and black pepper, then add this mixture to the potato ham mixture and mix well.
7. Line baking molds with parchment paper and pour in the tortilla mix.
8. Place the filled baking molds in the oven and bake until golden at the top.
9. Remove from the oven and let it cool. Remove from the mold, peel away the paper, and place on a serving plate.
10. Top with the queso fresco and parsley.

Fruity Yogurt Popsicles

Time: 4 hours and 5 minutes

Serving Size: 6

Prep Time: 5 minutes

Freeze Time: 4 hours

Ingredients:

- 1 cup nonfat plain Greek yogurt
- ½ cup skim milk
- ½ cup oats
- 1 cup chopped fruit

Directions:

1. Blend the yogurt and milk together.
2. Add the oats and mix well.
3. Sprinkle the fruit into the mixture and mix well.
4. Pour the mixture into the popsicle molds.
5. Place an ice cream stick in the middle of the mold.
6. Freeze the popsicles for at least 4 hours.

Peanut Butter and Jelly Pancakes

Time: 20 minutes

Serving Size: 4

Prep Time: 10 minutes

Cook Time: 10 minutes

Ingredients:

- 4 large egg whites
- ½ cup cottage cheese
- 2 tbsp powdered peanuts
- ½ cup oatmeal
- 1 cup mixed berry blend
- Butter

Directions:

1. In a blender, combine the egg whites, cottage cheese, powdered peanuts, and oatmeal and blend until smooth to make the batter.
2. Pour the mixture into a bowl, then fold in the mixed berry blend.
3. Grease the pan with a little bit of butter.
4. Pour ⅓ cup of batter on a pan and flip over once small bubbles at the top form, which will take about 3 minutes. Then cook for another 1 to 2 minutes. Repeat until you run out of batter.

Chapter 4: Solid Food Recipes– Lunch

Poultry Dishes

Cheesy Chicken Enchilada Soup

This cheesy and thick soup is so filling, it can stand alone as your main course. The thickness of the soup comes from the addition of the masa harina. Masa harina is a corn flour you can get from the grocery store in the flour section. This flour gives your soup an added corn flavor and a thickness to its consistency. This flour is the same kind used when making corn tortillas.

As for the cheese in this recipe, you should opt for block cheese and shred it before adding to the soup. Block cheeses melt better than pre-shredded ones, since those contain a coating that makes them not melt as well as freshly shredded cheeses.

Canned enchilada sauce can work for this recipe, but if you want to really make it flavorful, look for any homemade enchilada sauce recipes online. Enchilada sauce is usually not very time consuming to make and much more flavorful than the canned versions.

Instead of chicken, you may substitute ground or chopped turkey. Or, if you want this to be vegan-friendly, substitute canned corn kernels for the chicken, vegetable broth instead of chicken broth, and vegan cheddar for the cheese (or eliminate the cheese altogether if you're not partial to vegan cheese).

Time: 20 minutes

Serving Size: 4

Prep Time: 5 minutes

Cook Time: 15 minutes

Ingredients:

- 2 tbsp avocado oil
- 1 small onion, diced
- 2 cloves garlic, minced
- ½ cup masa harina
- 3 cups chicken broth
- ½ tsp ground cumin
- 2 cups chicken, cooked and shredded
- 1 tsp salt + salt to taste
- 1 ¼ cups enchilada sauce
- 1 15-ounce can of black beans, rinsed and drained
- 1 15-ounce can of diced tomatoes with juice
- 8 ounces cheddar cheese, grated

Directions:

1. Over medium high heat, heat the oil in a pot. Once the oil is hot, saute the onion until translucent, about 3 minutes.
2. Add the garlic and saute until fragrant, about 1 minute.

3. Add the masa harina and stir, letting it cook for 1 minute.

4. Add the chicken broth and mix well.

5. Add the cumin, chicken, salt, enchilada sauce, black beans, and tomatoes. Combine well. Stir occasionally and let the soup simmer. Reduce the heat to medium low.

6. Let the soup simmer for another 3 minutes, occasionally stirring. Add the cheese and stir until the cheese has melted and combined into the soup. Season with salt, if needed.

Cream of Chicken Soup

When needing something comforting, try this low-carb soup that's full of nutritious vegetables. You may also add or substitute any of your favorite vegetables in this soup and it would still be delicious.

To add flavor to the soup, if you have some time and have some chicken bones on hand, make chicken stock and keep it in the freezer. You can then add the chicken stock, which is more flavorful, instead of the canned version.

You can make a big batch of this soup, let it cool, then place in freezer containers and place in your freezer. When you want to eat the soup, let it thaw in the refrigerator overnight, then reheat over the stove or microwave.

For a lower-fat version of this soup, instead of using cream, you may use low-fat evaporated milk instead. Using evaporated milk also lets you store this soup in your freezer for months, without the broth curdling from the cream.

Time: 30 minutes

Serving Size: 6

Prep Time: 15 minutes

Cook Time: 15 minutes

Ingredients:

- 2 tsp olive oil
- 2 carrots, diagonally sliced
- 2 celery stalks, thinly sliced

- 1 leek, sliced into short, thin strips
- 4 tbsps butter
- ⅓ cup flour, sifted
- 6 cups chicken broth
- ⅓ cup cream

Directions:

1. Over medium heat, heat oil in a saucepan. Once the oil is hot, add the carrot, celery, and leek and cook until soft, about 6 to 7 minutes. Take the vegetables out of the pot and set aside.
2. Melt butter in the saucepan then add the flour and cook for 1 minute. Slowly stir in the broth and cream. Keep stirring until the soup boils.
3. Put the cooked vegetables back and add the chicken.

Avocado Egg Salad

This is a classic egg salad with the twist of adding mashed avocado. The mayonnaise keeps the salad moist, but it's not necessary to have if you don't like mayonnaise. Or, you can swap out the mayo with low-fat, plain yogurt.

Make this a hearty salad by keeping the ingredients chunky, so it's heftier to bite into. You can eat it on toasted bread, wrapped in a tortilla, lettuce, or collard, or top it onto your favorite salad.

To make the perfect hard boiled eggs, fill the pot with enough water to sit an inch above the eggs. Once the water starts boiling, turn off the heat, and let the eggs sit in the hot water for about 12 minutes. Cool off the eggs with cold water, so they don't get overcooked, and peeling the shell doesn't become difficult.

Time: 20 minutes

Serving Size: 2

Prep Time: 5 minutes

Cook Time: 15 minutes

Ingredients:

- 1 ½ tsp lemon juice
- 2 tbsp mayonnaise
- 1 medium avocado, peeled and pitted
- 1 tbsp chives, chopped
- 3 tbsp celery, finely chopped

- 4 hard-boiled eggs, peeled and chopped
- Salt and pepper

Directions:

1. Mash lemon juice, mayonnaise, and avocado in a bowl.
2. Add in the chives, celery, and eggs and combine well.
3. Add salt and pepper.

Pork and Beef Dishes

Pulled Pork

This pulled pork recipe is so tender and flavorful, you won't even need to put barbecue sauce on it anymore!

The best pork to use for this is a 4 to 7 pound pork shoulder that has a layer of fat at the bottom. There should be a bone going through the pork shoulder halfway through.

You will need a roasting pan that is 3 inches deep and big enough so that there is an inch of extra room on all sides of the pork. You also need a bag big enough to brine the pork in. Brining the pork gives it additional moisture, so it doesn't dry out while it's slow cooking.

Lastly, having a digital thermometer with an alarm will be a godsend for this dish. Since the pork takes such a long time to cook, it helps to have an alarm go off when the pork reaches a specific temperature. That way, you won't need to keep checking on the temperature.

Before seasoning the pork with the dry rub, pat it dry with paper towels so that when it cooks, the skin comes out with a crust.

To make the pork tender, we need to get the internal temperature of the pork to 200°F. Don't worry; since you've brined the pork, it won't dry out even when the temperature reaches up to 200°F.

Since this takes so long to cook, it's best to brine the pork two days before serving. Then that evening, season the pork with the dry rub and let the pork cook in the oven overnight. It will take at least 10 hours to cook.

When the alarm goes off in your digital thermometer, turn off the oven, but leave the pork in the oven for 2 more hours before taking it out. Leave in the thermometer so you can still check the temperature.

Check the pan. If it is dry, cover the pan with aluminum foil for the remaining 2 hours, so that the pork doesn't dry out.

Once the temperature drops down to 170°F, you may take the pork out of the oven.

Remove the layer of fat on the pork, then start pulling it apart. You may season the pork with the leftover dry rub if needed.

Time: 24 hours

Serving Size: 3 pounds

Prep Time: 12 hours

Cook Time: 12 hours

Ingredients:

- 4 to 7 pound whole pork shoulder, with a layer of fat, and bone-in
- ½ cup brown sugar + ½ cup
- 1 tbsp ground cumin
- 1 tbsp garlic powder
- 1 tbsp ground pepper

- 1 tbsp onion powder
- 1 tbsp salt + ½ cup
- 2 quarts of cold water
- 2 bay leaves

Directions:

1. For your dry rub, mix ½ cup brown sugar, cumin, garlic powder, ground pepper, onion powder, and 1 tbsp salt in an airtight container.

2. For your brine solution, dissolve the ½ cup salt in the cold water then add the bay leaves, 3 tbsp of dry rub, and ½ cup brown sugar and mix well.

3. Rinse the pork and put in a large container. Completely cover the pork with the brine solution. Cover the container, place in the refrigerator, and let the pork marinate in the brine solution for at least 12 hours.

4. After the pork is done marinating, preheat the oven to 225°F.

5. Take out the pork from the brine solution and pat dry with paper towels.

6. Place the pork in a baking pan that is at least 3 inches deep and at least an inch wider than the pork in width.

7. Massage the dry rub on the pork, making sure to coat all sides.

8. Position the pork facing fat up on the pan and insert a meat thermometer in the thickest part of the pork but not touching the bone. Place the pan in the middle rack of your oven.

9. Once the pork has reached 200°F, turn off the oven and let the roast cool in the oven for 2 hours before taking it out. Check the bottom of the pan. If it is dry, cover the pan with aluminum foil so the pork doesn't dry out while it cools. Once the pork has reached 170°F, take it out of the oven.

10. Place on a cutting board, remove the fat at the top, and pull the pork meat apart.

Asian Pork Tenderloin

Time: 1 day 50 minutes

Serving Size: 8

Prep Time: 1 day 10 minutes

Cook Time: 40 minutes

Ingredients:

- 4 garlic cloves, minced
- ⅓ cup light soy sauce
- 1 ½ tsp black pepper
- ⅓ cup brown sugar
- 1 tbsp ginger, minced
- 2 tbsp Worcestershire sauce
- 1 tbsp dry mustard
- 2 tbsp lemon juice
- 2 tbsp rice vinegar
- 2 pounds pork tenderloin

Directions:

1. Combine garlic, soy sauce, pepper, brown sugar, ginger, Worcestershire sauce, dry mustard, lemon juice, and rice vinegar in a bowl and mix well.
2. Place the pork in a freezer-safe bag and pour in the marinade. Rub the marinade on the meat.

3. Marinate the pork overnight in the refrigerator.
4. Preheat the oven to 375°F.
5. Bake the pork for 30 to 40 minutes.

Fish and Seafood Dishes

Avocado Tuna Salad Sandwich

Instead of using mayonnaise for this dish, we use avocado to keep it creamy. The lemon juice gives the salad that fresh, tangy flavor, while the celery and onion adds the contrasting crunch.

Make sure the avocado you get is ripe, so it's soft and easy to mash with a fork. Avocados that are ripe have a little give to it when you squeeze it.

You may need to season this a little bit more with salt and pepper since mayonnaise normally comes seasoned.

This is a salad that doesn't keep well for long, since it uses avocados. Avocados turn brown fairly quickly. If you don't mind eating it a little brown, you can keep it in the fridge for a few hours before consuming.

Time: 10 minutes

Serving Size: 2

Prep Time: 10 minutes

Cook Time: 0 minutes

Ingredients:

- 2 tbsp cilantro, chopped
- 1 5-ounce can of tuna in olive oil, drained
- 1 tsp lemon zest

- ½ avocado, chopped
- 2 tsp lemon juice
- ½ cup celery, minced
- 1 tbsp extra virgin olive oil
- ⅓ cup onion, minced
- Salt and pepper
- Bread

Directions:

1. Combine the avocado and tuna in a bowl and mash with a fork.
2. Add the rest of the ingredients and toss until all ingredients are well combined.
3. Season with salt and pepper.
4. Spread on bread.

Apple and Tuna Sandwich

Time: 15 minutes

Serving Size: 3

Prep Time: 15 minutes

Cook Time: 0 minutes

Ingredients:

- ½ tsp honey
- 1 6.5-ounce can tuna in water, drained
- 1 tsp mustard
- 1 Granny Smith apple, washed, peeled, and sliced into small pieces
- ¼ cup plain yogurt
- 6 slices whole wheat bread
- 3 lettuce leaves, washed

Directions:

1. Combine the honey, tuna, mustard, apple, and yogurt in a bowl and mix well.
2. Smear about ½ cup of the tuna spread on 3 slices of bread.
3. Put the lettuce on top, then add another slice of bread.

Vegetarian Dishes

Roasted Garlic Potato Soup

Roasting garlic makes the flavor mild and sweet, making it a perfect addition to a creamy potato soup. Roasted garlic is so versatile that it should be a staple in your kitchen. You can roast a bunch of garlic over the weekend and just store it for later.

This is a kind of soup that is a breeze to make, even during a weeknight. Just keep roasted garlic on hand, and add to the potato soup. This would take just about half an hour to make.

Time: 1 hour

Serving Size: 4

Prep Time: 10 minutes

Cook Time: 50 minutes

Ingredients:

- 1 head of garlic
- Olive oil
- Salt and pepper
- ¼ cup coconut oil mixed with a little bit of water
- 1 cup onions, chopped
- ¼ cup flour
- ¼ tsp thyme

- 4 cups vegetable broth
- ¼ cup soy milk with a little bit olive oil
- 1 cup almond milk
- ½ cup vegan parmesan cheese, grated
- 3 to 4 medium potatoes, peeled and boiled

Directions:

1. Preheat the oven to 375°F.
2. Peel a head of garlic, wet with some olive oil, and sprinkle with salt and pepper. Wrap with aluminum foil and place on a baking pan. Place the pan on a rack that is positioned in the middle of the oven. Roast the garlic for 40 to 45 minutes. Set aside to cool.
3. Over medium heat, in a large pot, pour in the coconut oil and water mixture. Once the oil is hot, sauté the onion until translucent, about 3 to 4 minutes.
4. Add the flour and cook for 1 minute, taking care not to burn the flour.
5. Add the thyme, broth, soy milk and olive oil mixture, almond milk, and salt and pepper. Mix well, let it come to a boil, then simmer for 2 to 3 minutes, stirring occasionally.
6. Add the vegan parmesan cheese, 8 or 9 roasted cloves of garlic, and the potatoes. Cook for a few minutes, then pour the soup in a blender and puree. Serve warm.

Tomato Soup

This soup is so easy to prepare, and it will be done in one hour. This dish is vegan, but for our non-vegan friends, adding some ham or bacon to this soup definitely adds a great smoky flavor that goes well with the soup.

This soup is best paired with some crunchy garlic toast to dunk in all that goodness.

Time: 1 hour

Serving Size: 4

Prep Time: 10 minutes

Cook Time: 50 minutes

Ingredients:

- 2 tbsp olive oil
- ½ onion, chopped
- 4 cloves garlic, minced
- 2 carrots, chopped
- 1 ½ tbsp tomato paste
- 1 tbsp flour
- 1 bay leaf
- 1 28-ounce can crushed tomatoes
- ½ tsp dried thyme
- 4 cups vegetable broth
- Salt and pepper

Directions:

1. Over medium low heat, heat olive oil. Once hot, sauté the onion until translucent, about 3 minutes.
2. Add the garlic and sauté until fragrant, about 1 minute.
3. Add the carrots and cook until tender, about 5 to 10 minutes.
4. Add the tomato paste and stir until the tomato paste starts to brown.
5. Add the flour and stir for 1 minute.
6. Add the bay leaf, crushed tomatoes, thyme, and broth. Let the soup simmer for 30 minutes.
7. Puree the soup and return to the pot. Season with salt and pepper.

Tomato, Basil, and Quinoa Salad With Vegan Mozzarella

This is a cold salad, packed with Italian flavors. It is filling, yet very light. The rice vinegar, salt and pepper, and olive oil adds a tang to the salad, while the vegan mozzarella adds a little creaminess with each bite. You can add any fresh produce you have on hand to this salad, and it will still be delicious. Amp up the nutrients in this salad by adding tempeh, zucchini, tofu, cucumber, summer squash, avocado, carrots, and bell peppers. If you don't have cherry or grape tomatoes on hand, you can add diced heirloom tomatoes.

You can also use other types of vegan cheese instead of mozzarella, and it will still work well. If you do not have quinoa on hand, you may use couscous or brown rice instead.

Before cooking the quinoa, make sure you rinse it well so it doesn't taste bitter.

If you make the salad a day before eating it, it will be more flavorful.

Time: 25 minutes

Serving Size: 4

Prep Time: 5 minutes

Cook Time: 20 minutes

Ingredients:

- 2 cups quinoa, cooked according to package instructions

- 3 tbsp olive oil
- 1 cup cherry or grape tomatoes
- 4 tbsp rice vinegar
- 1 cup vegan mozzarella cheese balls
- Basil leaves to taste
- ¼ tsp sugar
- Salt and pepper

Directions:

1. Combine the quinoa, olive oil, tomatoes, rice vinegar, vegan mozzarella, and basil leaves in a bowl.
2. Season with sugar, salt, and pepper.

Chapter 5: Solid Food Recipes– Dinner

Poultry Dishes

Couscous Chicken Soup

When you're feeling under the weather, what is better than having a bowl of chicken soup? This recipe is as comforting as the soup mom makes. This soup has lemongrass, ginger, turmeric, lemon, and garlic, all ingredients that are good for your health.

If you want to freeze this soup and keep it in stock, you can make the soup base, let it cool, and freeze that. The couscous does not freeze well, however, so you will have to cook that separately and add to the heated soup when you're about to eat it.

If you're in a hurry, you can substitute instant rice instead of couscous, which cooks faster.

Time: 35 minutes

Serving Size: 4

Prep Time: 15 minutes

Cook Time: 20 minutes

Ingredients:

- 4 cups chicken broth

- ½ cup celery, chopped
- 1 cup onions, chopped
- ½ cup carrots, sliced
- ¾ cup leeks, sliced
- 2 cloves garlic, minced
- 1 tbsp lemongrass, minced
- 1 tbsp ginger, minced
- ½ tsp ground turmeric
- 1 cup couscous
- 8 ounces chicken, cooked and shredded
- Juice from ½ lemon
- Salt and pepper

Directions:

1. Over medium heat, pour one tablespoon of the chicken broth in a pot. Once the broth is sizzling, sauté the celery, onions, carrots, and leeks until soft, about 6 minutes.
2. Add the garlic, lemongrass, and ginger and sauté until fragrant. Then, add the turmeric and combine well.
3. Add the couscous, chicken, and broth, and bring the soup to a boil.
4. Lower the heat and let the soup simmer for 15 minutes. Season with the lemon, salt, and pepper.

Chicken with Peanut Applesauce

Time: 1 hour and 10 minutes

Serving Size: 8

Prep Time: 10 minutes

Cook Time: 1 hour

Ingredients:

- 2 ½ pounds chicken, cut into serving pieces
- ½ cup powdered peanuts
- 1 15-ounce jar unsweetened applesauce
- ⅛ cup brown sugar
- ¼ cup yellow mustard

Directions:

1. Over medium low heat, cook chicken in a pan for about 13 to 15 minutes.
2. Once almost fully cooked, add the peanuts, applesauce, brown sugar, and mustard and mix all ingredients together.
3. Let the ingredients simmer over medium heat until the chicken reaches an internal temperature of at least 165°F.

Baked Chicken and Vegetables

Time: 1 hour and 15 minutes

Serving Size: 6

Prep Time: 15 minutes

Cook Time: 1 hour

Ingredients:

- 1 onion, quartered
- 6 carrots, sliced
- 4 potatoes, sliced
- 1 skinless chicken, cut into serving pieces
- ¼ tsp pepper
- 1 tsp thyme
- ½ cup water

Directions:

1. Preheat the oven to 400°F.
2. Arrange the onions, carrots, and potatoes in a roasting pan.
3. Place the chicken on top of the vegetables.
4. In a bowl, mix pepper, thyme, and water. Pour this mixture over the chicken and vegetables.
5. Bake the chicken until browned, for about an hour.
6. Baste the chicken sporadically while it is baking.

Pork and Beef Dishes

Shepherd's Pie

This classic dish is composed of gravy, pot roast, cheese, and mashed potatoes. You may use your favorite mashed potato recipe for this, or leftover mashed potatoes if you have any on hand. If you don't have a recipe, there is a mashed potato recipe available in this book that you can use (Creamy Garlic Herb Mashed Potatoes).

Time: 7 hours and 25 minutes

Serving Size: 4

Prep Time: 15 minutes

Cook Time: 7 hours and 10 minutes

Ingredients:

- 2 pounds pot roast
- 1 cup carrots, shredded
- ¼ tsp pepper
- 1 cup beef broth
- 1 tsp oregano
- 3 beef bouillon cubes + 2 beef smashed bouillon cubes
- 2 tbsp cumin
- 3 tbsp garlic, minced
- ¼ cup butter

- ¼ cup flour
- 3 cups milk
- 1 cup peas
- 6 cups mashed potatoes (use your favorite mashed potato recipe)
- 1 cup cheddar cheese, shredded

Directions:

1. Preheat the oven to 350°F.
2. Place roast in a slow cooker with carrots, beef broth, oregano, 3 bouillon cubes, cumin, garlic, and cayenne pepper.
3. Cook on high for 4 to 6 hours.
4. Once cooked, slice the roast into bite-sized pieces.
5. Over medium heat, melt butter in a saucepan.
6. Add flour and cook for 1 minute.
7. Add the 2 smashed beef bouillon cubes and milk.
8. Stir until the gravy boils and thickens.
9. In a 9x13 inch baking dish, layer the roast at the bottom of the baking dish, followed by the peas, gravy, and finally, cover with the mashed potatoes.
10. Place the baking dish in the oven and bake for 50 to 60 minutes.
11. Remove from the oven and sprinkle with cheese on top. Return to the oven and bake until the cheese melts, about 5 minutes.

Pork and Black Bean Stew

Time: 1 hour 30 minutes

Serving Size: 4

Prep Time: 15 minutes

Cook Time: 1 hour 15 minutes

Ingredients:

- 1 tsp ground black pepper
- 1 tbsp ground coriander
- 1 tsp onion powder
- 1 tbsp ground cumin
- 2 tsp oregano
- 1 tbsp ground annatto
- 1 tbsp salt
- 1 tbsp garlic powder
- 2 tsp extra-virgin olive oil
- 1 pound pork tenderloin, fat trimmed and sliced into 1 inch cubes
- 1 ¼ cup onions, chopped
- 3 garlic cloves
- 1 14.5-ounce can unsalted black beans, rinsed and drained
- 1 14.5-ounce can tomatoes with juice

- 1 14-ounce can unsalted chicken broth

Directions:

1. Make the spice blend by combining the black pepper, ground coriander, onion powder, cumin, oregano, annatto, salt, and garlic powder in an airtight container and mixing well.
2. Over medium high heat, heat olive oil in a pot. Once the oil is hot, cook the pork until brown, about 4 to 6 minutes.
3. Add the onion and sauté until translucent, about 3 minutes.
4. Add the garlic and sauté until fragrant, about 1 minute.
5. Add 1 ½ tsp of spice mix and stir.
6. Add the beans, tomatoes, and broth and stir.
7. Bring the stew to a boil then lower heat.
8. Cover and let the stew simmer until the pork is tender, about 45 minutes to 1 hour.
9. Serve with rice.

Fish and Seafood Dishes

Pan-Fried Trout

Time: 25 minutes

Serving Size: 2

Prep Time: 10 minutes

Cook Time: 15 minutes

Ingredients:

- 8 ounces trout fillets
- 1 ⅓ tbsp parsley, chopped
- 3 tbsp cornmeal
- ¼ tsp ground celery seeds
- 1 pinch salt
- ¼ tsp ground black pepper
- 2 tsp olive oil

Directions:

1. Clean and rinse the fish, checking for and removing any bones. Pat dry with paper towels.
2. Mix chopped parsley, cornmeal, celery seed, salt, and pepper in a bowl.
3. Coat the fish with the cornmeal mix.

4. Heat the olive oil in a pan. When the oil is very hot, place the fish in the pan and cook until the fish is brown and crisp and is flakey, about 2 to 3 minutes on each side.

Shrimp Ceviche

Time: 25 minutes

Serving Size: 4

Prep Time: 25 minutes

Cook Time: 0 minutes

Ingredients:

- 1 cup lime juice
- 1 pound raw shrimp, peeled and deveined
- 1 bunch cilantro, stems removed and finely chopped
- 1 onion, finely chopped
- ½ medium green bell pepper, minced
- 4 medium tomatoes, diced
- Salt

Directions:

1. Combine lime juice and shrimp in a bowl.
2. Cover and let the shrimp marinate until the color changes to pink, about 10 to 15 minutes. Do not let the shrimp marinate too long or it will become tough.
3. Add cilantro, onion, bell pepper, tomatoes.
4. Season with salt.
5. Serve cold.

Vegetarian Dishes

Vegetarian Fried Rice

This fried rice is overloaded with vegetables, and it's so filling, it can stand as a main dish on its own! To change this up, you can add or substitute your favorite vegetables with the ones in the recipe. You may also use fresh or frozen vegetables in this recipe. For non-vegetarians looking for meat, you may add some cooked, diced chicken breasts.

This dish calls for a lot of chopping, so if you have a vegetable chopper on hand, it's time to break it out. Other than all the chopping, everything else is fairly simple.

This dish works best if you use day old rice from the refrigerator, as this kind of rice tends to be drier and can absorb the sauce better. If you do not have day old rice on hand, don't fret. Freshly cooked rice works as well, but let it cool first before adding it to the wok, and let it cook in the wok for a longer time, so that the rice dries out.

Time: 20 minutes

Serving Size: 4

Prep Time: 5 minutes

Cook Time: 15 minutes

Ingredients:

- 2 tbsp canola oil
- 1 cup yellow onions, chopped

- 4 cloves garlic, minced
- 1 tbsp fresh ginger, minced
- 1 cup carrots, diced thinly
- ¾ cup red bell pepper, diced into small pieces
- 1 ½ cups broccoli, diced into small pieces
- 4 large eggs
- 1 tbsp sesame oil
- 3 cups cooked, chilled white rice
- Soy sauce to taste
- ¾ cup frozen peas, thawed and drained
- ¾ cup frozen baby corn, thawed and drained

Directions:

1. On medium-high heat, heat oil in a wok or a deep pan. When the oil is hot, saute the onions until translucent, about 3 minutes.
2. Add the garlic and saute until fragrant, about 1 minute.
3. Add the ginger and carrots and saute for 3 minutes.
4. Add the bell pepper and broccoli and saute until desired tenderness, about 3-4 minutes. Move all the vegetables to one side of the pan.
5. On the opposite side of the vegetables, crack the eggs, scramble, and cook through. Once cooked, mix the eggs with the vegetables.
6. Add the sesame oil, rice, soy sauce, peas, and corn. Toss for 2 minutes.

Roasted Root Vegetables

Time: 1 hour 5 minutes

Serving Size: 6

Prep Time: 25 minutes

Cook Time: 40 minutes

Ingredients:

- ¼ tsp salt
- Black pepper
- ⅓ cup cider vinegar
- 3 tbsp brown sugar
- ½ cup extra virgin olive oil
- 1 large onion, sliced thickly
- 4 medium beets, peeled and sliced thickly
- 4 medium parsnips, peeled and sliced into 2-inch long pieces
- 4 medium carrots, peeled and sliced into 2-inch long pieces
- 3 medium yams, sliced into 2-inch long pieces
- ¾ tsp thyme

Directions:

1. Preheat the oven to 450°F.

2. Combine the salt, pepper, cider vinegar, brown sugar, and olive oil with the onion, beets, parsnips, carrots, and yams in a bowl.

3. Line sheet pans with aluminum foil and spread out the vegetables in the pan. Drizzle the leftover vinaigrette dressing in the bowl over the vegetables.

4. Roast the vegetables in the oven until the vegetables have browned and caramelized, about 35 to 40 minutes. Halfway through roasting, turn the pans and switch from bottom to top rack positions.

5. Once roasted, take the sheet pans out of the oven and sprinkle the vegetables with thyme, and salt, and pepper to taste.

Vegetarian Chili

Time: 50 minutes

Serving Size: 10

Prep Time: 10 minutes

Cook Time: 40 minutes

Ingredients:

- 1 tbsp peanut oil
- 1 cup onion, chopped
- 2 cloves garlic, minced
- Salt and pepper
- ¼ tsp oregano
- 2 cups vegetable broth
- 1 16-ounce can white beans, rinsed and drained
- 1 16-ounce can black beans, rinsed and drained
- 1 15-ounce can tomato sauce
- 1 28-ounce can tomatoes, diced
- ⅔ cup powdered peanuts

Directions:

1. Over medium high heat, heat oil in a pan. Once the oil is hot, saute the onion until translucent, about 3 minutes.
2. Add the garlic and saute until fragrant, about 1 minute.

3. Mix in the salt, pepper, and oregano and saute for 2 more minutes.
4. Add the broth, beans, tomato sauce, tomatoes, and powdered peanuts, and bring to a boil.
5. Lower the heat and let it simmer for 30 minutes.

Chapter 6: Solid Food Recipes– Snacks, Sides, Desserts

Snacks

Cheesy Potato and Turkey Pancakes

With this dish, you can use any of your favorite mashed potato recipes. Should you not have one, the one in this book will work perfectly (Creamy Garlic Herb Mashed Potatoes). If you're using leftover mashed potatoes for this recipe, the consistency will vary depending on how much butter, milk, and cream were used when the mashed potatoes were made. If it is looking too dry, add an egg. If it is too wet, add one tablespoon of flour to dry it out and make it stickier.

Time: 25 minutes

Serving Size: 12 pancakes

Prep Time: 20 minutes

Cook Time: 5 minutes

Ingredients:

- 3 tbsp flour
- 3 cups chilled mashed potatoes
- 1 egg, beaten
- ⅔ cup cheese, shredded
- ½ cup turkey, chopped
- 2 tbsp scallions, chopped + additional scallions for topping

- Vegetable oil
- Sour cream for topping

Directions:

1. Combine 3 tbsp flour, mashed potatoes, egg, cheese, turkey, and scallions in a bowl.
2. Divide the mixture into 12 compact balls then flatten into a ½-inch thick pancake.
3. Dredge each pancake with the ½ cup flour.
4. Over medium heat, heat oil in a frying pan (enough to coat the bottom of the pan).
5. Fry the pancakes in batches until they are crispy and golden brown on both sides, about 3 to 4 minutes. Make sure that the pancakes are not overcrowded in the pan when frying, and that you don't flip them over too soon, so they develop a crispy crust.
6. Once cooked, place on a plate lined with paper towels to absorb the excess oil. Sprinkle with salt, if needed, immediately after taking out of the pan.
7. You may add more oil in the pan if needed between batches.
8. Top with scallions and sour cream before serving.

Quinoa Fruit Salad With Honey Lemon Dressing

This is such a fresh, light summer salad. The quinoa not only adds texture to the salad, but it's healthy and chock full of vitamins, minerals, and protein as well. The honey lemon dressing gives a little tang to the fruits.

Before cooking the quinoa, make sure you rinse it well so it doesn't taste bitter.

Time: 20 minutes

Serving Size: 6

Prep Time: 20 minutes

Cook Time: 0 minutes

Ingredients:

- 1 mango, diced
- 1 cup quinoa, cooked according to the package instructions
- 1 ½ cup strawberries, sliced
- 1 cup blueberries
- 1 cup blackberries
- ¼ cup honey
- 2 tbsp lime juice
- 1 tbsp basil, chopped

Directions:

1. Combine the mango, quinoa, strawberries, blueberries, and blackberries in a bowl.
2. In a separate bowl, mix the honey and lime juice together, then pour over the fruit mix and toss.
3. Sprinkle with basil.

Apple Zucchini Bread

This is a bread that is crumbly and a little crispy on the outside, but moist and dense on the inside. It has a hint of apple flavor to it, which is complemented by the nutmeg and cinnamon.

When taking the bread out of the pan, loosen the edges of the bread with a butter knife so that you can easily take it out of the pan.

This bread is best eaten for breakfast or as a snack with your tea, coffee, or even apple cider. You may also spread a little bit of butter to add to the flavor.

Time: 1 hour 30 minutes

Serving Size: 1 loaf

Prep Time: 30 minutes

Cook Time: 60 minutes

Ingredients:

- ½ tsp nutmeg
- 2 cups all-purpose flour
- ½ tbsp baking soda
- 1 tsp ground cinnamon
- ¼ tsp salt
- 2 large eggs
- ½ tbsp vanilla extract
- ¾ cup olive oil

- ½ cup brown sugar
- 1 cup white sugar
- ¾ cup pecans, chopped
- ½ cup apple, peeled and shredded
- 1 cup zucchini, unpeeled and shredded

Directions:

1. Preheat the oven to 350°F.
2. Combine nutmeg, flour, baking soda, cinnamon, and salt in a bowl.
3. In a separate bowl, beat the eggs, then add the vanilla, oil, brown sugar, and white sugar. Mix well and pour over the dry mix. Combine well.
4. Add in the pecans, apples, and zucchini.
5. Transfer the batter to a greased and floured 8x4-inch loaf pan.
6. Bake until a toothpick inserted in the middle of the loaf comes out clean, about 55 to 60 minutes.
7. Once the bread is done baking, take out of the oven and let it sit in the pan for 15 minutes. Then take the loaf out of the pan and let it completely cool on a wire rack.

Blueberry Sour Cream Cake

Time: 55 minutes

Serving Size: 16 servings

Prep Time: 10 minutes

Cook Time: 45 minutes

Ingredients:

- 2 cups white sugar
- 1 cup butter, softened
- 2 eggs
- 1 tsp vanilla extract
- 1 cup sour cream
- ¼ tsp salt
- 1 tsp baking powder
- 1 ¾ cups all-purpose flour
- 1 ½ cups blueberries
- ½ cup pecans, chopped
- 1 tsp ground cinnamon
- ½ cup brown sugar
- Confectioners' sugar

Directions:

1. Preheat the oven to 350°F.

2. Mix the sugar and butter in a bowl until light and fluffy. Add the eggs and beat one at a time, then mix in the vanilla and sour cream. Be careful not to overmix the batter, as this will cause your cake to deflate.

3. In a separate bowl, combine the salt, baking powder, and flour. Blend this with the batter, then fold in the blueberries.

4. In another bowl, combine the pecans, cinnamon, and brown sugar. Set aside.

5. Grease and flour a 9-inch Bundt pan.

6. Pour half of the batter into the greased Bundt pan then sprinkle with the pecan mixture. Pour the rest of the batter into the pan and sprinkle the rest of the pecan mixture on top. Take a knife and swirl the batter.

7. Bake until a knife inserted into the cake's crown comes out clean, about 50 to 60 minutes.

8. Once baked, take it out of the oven and let it cool completely. Invert and tap the Bundt pan over a serving plate to remove the cake. Drizzle with confectioners' sugar.

Sides

Mashed Cauliflower and Sweet Potatoes

Sweet potatoes aren't just for thanksgiving. With this easy recipe, you can make them any time you're craving for them. They are the perfect healthy food for those looking for something filling and nutritious to go along with their main dishes.

Time: 27 minutes

Serving Size: 4

Prep Time: 15 minutes

Cook Time: 12 minutes

Ingredients:

- 1 pound cauliflower florets
- 2 pounds sweet potatoes, peeled and sliced into 1 ½-inch chunks
- 3 tbsp milk
- ½ tsp garlic powder
- ¼ cup plain Greek yogurt
- Salt and pepper
- Fresh parsley, chopped

Directions:

1. Steam the cauliflower and sweet potato until tender, for 10 to 12 minutes.
2. With the milk, mash the cauliflower and sweet potato in a bowl. Mix in the garlic powder and Greek yogurt. Add salt and pepper to taste. To thin out the mixture if needed, add more milk 1 tbsp at a time to your desired consistency.
3. Sprinkle chopped parsley on top.

Ham and Egg Baked Potato Bowls

This dish is so delicious and filling, with the egg, potato, ham, and cheese—it could be a snack on its own!

The potatoes will be cooked in the oven. To see if they're cooked through, run a butter knife through the center of the potato. If it runs through smoothly with hardly any resistance, it means the potato is cooked through.

You will need to scoop out the potato to make a bowl. You can use the scooped out potatoes to make mashed potatoes. There is a recipe in this book for Creamy Garlic Herb Mashed Potatoes that you can use.

These potato bowls are excellent with a garlic yogurt dip. You just need some low fat yogurt, combined with some minced garlic, a little bit of lemon juice, and some salt to taste.

Time: 1 hour 20 minutes

Serving Size: 3

Prep Time: 10 minutes

Cook Time: 1 hour 10 minutes

Ingredients:

- 6 large potatoes
- 3 tbsp olive oil
- Salt and pepper
- 5 ounces cheese, shredded
- 6 eggs

- 2 stalks green onions, chopped
- 9 ounces ham, cubed

Directions:

1. Preheat the oven to 400°F.
2. Wash and brush the potatoes thoroughly under running water.
3. Place the potatoes in the oven and bake until they are cooked and soft inside, about 40 minutes.
4. Take the potatoes out of the oven and set aside to cool.
5. Lower the oven heat to 350°F.
6. When the potatoes are cool enough to handle by hand, slice the top layer off each potato and scoop out the insides. Do not tear or puncture the bottom of the potatoes.
7. Coat the inside of the potato with oil and season with salt and pepper.
8. Fill the inside of each potato halfway with cheese, green onions, and ham.
9. Crack an egg in each potato.
10. Add more cheese, green onions, and ham to the potato until filled to the top, and season with more salt and pepper.
11. Place the potatoes back in the oven and bake until the egg whites have set, for about 20 minutes.

Cauliflower and Cheddar Cheese Bake

This side dish is loaded with flavor from the cream cheese, ham, and cheddar cheese, but low on carbs. You may use either fresh or frozen cauliflowers. After cooking the cauliflower and adding the cream cheese and butter, the easiest way to mash it would be to use a hand mixer, and mix it to your desired consistency.

Time: 1 hour

Serving Size: 4

Prep Time: 30 minutes

Cook Time: 30 minutes

Ingredients:

- Salt
- 2 medium size cauliflower heads
- ½ cup of butter
- 8 ounces plain cream cheese
- 4 ½ ounces ham, cooked and chopped
- Green onions, chopped
- 1 ¼ cups cheddar cheese, shredded
- Pepper

Directions:

1. Preheat the oven to 350°F.

2. Sprinkle salt in some water and boil the cauliflower in it until soft. Drain the water, then return the cauliflower to the pot.

3. Add the butter and cream cheese to the pot and mash to desired consistency.

4. Scoop into a baking dish and top with the ham, green onions, and cheese. Sprinkle with a little salt and pepper.

5. Place the dish in the oven and bake for 20 to 30 minutes.

Desserts

Apple Carrot Bread

This bread is sweet and perfect for dessert. It is light, soft, moist, tender, but still dense and satisfying. It tastes like carrot cake with a hint of apple. The carrots and apples together make this bread sweet and moist.

Any kind of apple will work for this recipe. To grate the apples and carrots, you can use the coarsest grate on a box grater or a food processor.

Before mixing the batter, let the egg and sour cream sit out for a little while, until they reach room temperature; that way, when you mix them in with the coconut oil, the oil doesn't re-solidify. Coconut oil has a tendency to re-solidify at the slightest cold, and if it does, you might end up with pools of oil in your batter.

If the sides and top of your bread are turning too brown while baking, place a sheet of aluminum foil draped loosely over the pan so that the center can cook through. Do not just rely on the baking times provided, as baking times differ depending on the oven, how much moisture the apples and carrots contain, and the climate.

We use coconut oil here instead of butter because coconut oil keeps the bread softer than butter does. Coconut oil also has a slightly sweeter flavor than other types of oils.

The batter will be very thick. It needs to be thick because as the apples and carrots bake, they release juices into the bread. If your batter is too watery, it will turn into soup when it bakes.

You can add a butter glaze to the bread to add to the flavor.

Time: 1 hour 10 minutes

Serving Size: 1 loaf

Prep Time: 25 minutes (including 15 minutes cooling time)

Cook Time: 45 minutes

Ingredients:

- ½ tsp ground nutmeg
- 1 large egg
- 2 tsp cinnamon
- ½ cup brown sugar
- 2 tsp vanilla extract
- ⅓ cup coconut oil
- ¼ cup sour cream
- ¼ cup granulated sugar
- Pinch of salt
- 1 cup all-purpose flour
- ½ tsp baking soda
- ½ tsp baking powder
- ¾ cup apples, grated
- ¾ cup carrots, grated

Directions:

1. Preheat the oven to 350°F.
2. Combine the first eight ingredients listed above (from ground nutmeg through granulated sugar), in a bowl.
3. Fold in the salt, flour, baking soda, and baking powder into the mixture. Do not overmix.
4. Add the apples and carrots and fold gently.
5. Put the batter in the greased and floured 9x5-inch loaf pan. Using a spatula, smooth the top.
6. Bake until a toothpick inserted in the middle of the bread comes out clean and the top is golden, about 45 to 52 minutes.
7. Once the bread is done, let it cool in the pan for 15 minutes before taking it out.

Vanilla Mug Cake

This cake is made in a mug and meant to be baked in a microwave. It is easy to make. This recipe does not contain any eggs, but the texture is the same as a full sized cake. You can use self-raising flour if you want the texture to be spongy. Using all purpose flour will make the cake moist, fluffy, and light.

For variety, you may opt to add other ingredients, such as peanut butter or nutella, to the cake before placing it in the microwave to bake, since the cake is a base flavor.

Time: 7 minutes

Serving Size: 1

Prep Time: 5 minutes

Cook Time: 2 minutes

Ingredients:

- 1/8 tsp salt
- ¼ cup all-purpose flour + 2 tbsp
- ¼ tsp baking powder
- 2 tbsp granulated sugar
- ½ tbsp vanilla extract
- 1 tsp vanilla bean paste
- 2 tbsp butter, melted

Directions:

1. Whisk the salt, flour, baking powder, and sugar in a bowl.
2. Mix the vanilla extract, vanilla bean paste, and milk in a separate bowl.
3. Make a crater in the middle of the dry ingredient mix and pour the wet ingredient mix in the middle, then pour the butter on top.
4. Mix until the batter is combined well and smooth, then pour the batter into a microwave-safe mug.
5. Microwave on high for 2 minutes and 10 seconds.

Sticky Lemon Cake

This cake is not too sweet and a little tart—a certain hit for those who like lemon-flavored pastries and desserts.

This cake is pretty straightforward to bake. You just need to cream the sugar and butter with the lemon zest, then add the yolk and eggs, then the yogurt and other dry ingredients. The yogurt lessens the sweetness of the cake and the almond flour makes it dense.

Use a baking pan that's 3 inches high to give the cake enough room to rise without spilling over the pan.

Time: 1 hour 10 minutes

Serving Size: 1 cake

Prep Time: 20 minutes

Cook Time: 50 minutes

Ingredients:

- Zest from 2 lemons
- ¾ cup sugar + ½ cup set aside
- 1 ½ sticks of butter
- 2 large eggs + 1 egg yolk
- 2 tsp baking powder
- ½ cups all-purpose flour
- 1 ⅓ cups almond flour
- 2 tbsp lemon juice + 4 tbsp set aside

- 1 ⅓ cups plain yogurt

Directions:

1. Preheat the oven to 325°F.
2. Combine the zest, ¾ cup sugar, and butter. Beat in the eggs, one by one.
3. Combine the baking powder, all-purpose flour, and almond flour in a separate bowl and mix well. Add to the butter mixture along with 2 tbsp of lemon juice and yogurt.
4. Grease an 8x3-inch cake pan and line the pan with parchment paper.
5. Pour the batter in the pan and bake until a toothpick inserted in the center of the cake comes out clean, about 45 to 50 minutes.
6. Over low heat, mix the remaining 4 tbsp lemon juice and ½ cup sugar in a saucepan until the sugar dissolves. Let it cool.
7. Once the cake is done baking, let it cool on a wire rack. Using a skewer, punch holes in the cake and drizzle with the lemon syrup. Let it cool for 30 minutes. Remove the cake from the pan then remove the parchment paper and let the cake cool completely.

Chapter 7: Tips When Dining Out

Dining out cannot be avoided nowadays, but until you've reached the solid food stage, it might be wise to have your meals prepared and eaten at home. This is wise, in part, because dining out might cause some anxiety, in the beginning, for you, because you might be afraid of eating the wrong foods or overeating. Instead of avoiding it, learn how to select the correct food. Be prepared though; dining out after you've had your gastric sleeve surgery is going to be very different compared to before!

People who have undergone bariatric procedures receive a Weight Loss Surgery card which will allow you to order a smaller portion of an entree in a restaurant at a discounted price. So when dining out, don't forget to bring this card!

Prior to going to the restaurant, take a look at the restaurant's menu and nutrition facts via the Internet, so you can check for the healthiest entree you can eat. Even the children's menu may not be the answer; while the portions may be smaller, the food is still full of fat and high in calories. Look for dishes high in protein first, then vegetables. Proteins should be lean proteins from chicken, fish, and turkey. You may have carbs, but keep to complex carbohydrates like whole wheat pasta and yams. Make it a point to check how many calories dishes have. Most restaurants will be able to provide you with the calorie content of their dishes.

Upon ordering, instruct the server to have your food prepared in a low-fat manner, to be baked or broiled and have no fat, oil, or butter added. Avoid food that is breaded, pan-fried, or fried. If needed, be assertive, and ask for an order to be customized to fit your dietary needs. Ask your server not to bring any bread baskets or chips to your table to lessen temptation. More often than not, the entree will be more than you can eat, so plan on bringing most of it home. Once your food is served, before you start eating, portion out the food to ½ cup vegetables, ¼ cup carbs, and 3 ounces of protein. Have the rest put in a take out box. Or, you can order one main course and split it with someone, or perhaps one or two appetizers instead of a main course. Don't feel that you need to finish all that food though! Eat until you are satisfied and have any leftovers put in the take out box.

Eat slowly and chew your food until it is liquid in consistency. Set your utensils down with each bite to help you slow down when you eat. <u>Do not drink anything while eating.</u> Drinking fluids while eating may push your food down and make you eat more. Refrain from drinking fluids 15 minutes prior to eating, and wait 30 minutes after eating before drinking.

You should not have alcohol for one full year after your surgery, and after that you can only have very small amounts. Alcohol is full of empty calories, and for those who have gone through bariatric surgery, your system absorbs alcohol quicker, making it more potent. There is also a chance of developing an ulcer when consuming alcohol regularly, as well as developing a dependency to it.

Most likely, you're dining out to socialize and be with other people, so mingle, catch up with friends, and cut a rug on the dance floor. Make conversation your focal point, instead of eating. Do more talking and listening to the conversation than eating. If you're at a party or a wedding, sit far away from the buffet table. Quickly scan the available food at the buffet table and make a plan on what food you will eat during the event. If it is a sit down dinner event and the food is being served, call the caterer ahead of time and ask what will be served, and make a request so the food served to you meets your dietary needs.

Chapter 8: How to Maintain Your Weight After Surgery

Gastric sleeve surgery is <u>not</u> the miracle cure to end obesity. It is a <u>tool</u> to help you lead a healthier life, and to do this, you will need to make permanent adjustments in your lifestyle. This includes the level of physical activity you do daily, your eating habits, how you manage stress, behaviors, and your mindset; all of these will need to be reevaluated in order for you to lose weight and keep the weight off. Create and maintain healthy habits to lead to a healthy life.

Establishing Healthy Eating Habits

Eat to Lose Weight

As counterintuitive as it may sound, it is important that you not starve yourself! Fuel your body with the right kinds of food, those high in lean protein and complex carbohydrates. To start your day off on the right foot, eat breakfast within 1 to 2 hours of waking up. Doing so helps your body maintain a stable blood sugar level throughout the day. Make a conscious effort not to skip meals, even if you feel like you're not hungry. Establish meal times and follow the schedule; do not go without eating while awake for more than 4 to 5 hours. Studies have shown that fasting, or not eating for prolonged periods of time, causes your body to produce more ghrelin, or hunger-inducing hormones, than normal. An increase in hunger may cause overeating on your part, which can also lead to extreme swings in your energy and blood sugar levels.

Meal Planning Is One of the Keys to Success

Plan your meals so it's easier to eat healthy instead of reaching for just whatever is available. To start meal planning, make a list of dishes you enjoy eating, including go-to dishes that are easy to prepare when in a rush. Protein shakes and powders are easy to prepare for breakfast or a snack if you're hungry and in a hurry, so it would be a good idea to keep this on hand at home.

Also, keep some canned vegetables at home for convenience. While fresh and frozen vegetables are more nutritious than canned vegetables, canned vegetables have fast food beat when it comes to being nutritious.

As much as possible, avoid eating out and prepare your own food at home so you know exactly what goes in the food you're eating.

What Should You Be Eating?

Protein is a very important macronutrient that you should include in your diet. However, not all proteins are the same. Stick to lean proteins such as soy products, fish, eggs, chicken, low-fat dairy, lean pork, and lean red meat.

Proteins such as cheese, pork sausages, bacon, salami, and prime rib are high in fat and shouldn't be consumed often.

Plant-based proteins are marketed as the healthier alternative, however, these do not have the essential amino acids that are beneficial to your body that animal-based proteins do. While the fat these plant-based proteins are usually good for your heart, since the fat content is very high, it may cause you to gain weight. Plant-based proteins are also usually high in carbohydrates and calories, so keep this in mind if you're looking to increase your protein intake.

Make small adjustments to your meals. For example, to keep your protein intake the same, but lower the fat, substitute with chicken when a recipe calls for beef.

Make the majority of the food you eat nutrient-dense, low-calorie food, such as fruits and vegetables. Fruits and vegetables fill you up faster without too many calories. You should be eating five servings of fruits and vegetables daily–three servings of non-starchy vegetables, and two servings of fruit. Work slowly up to this amount by starting out with just one serving of fruit and one serving of vegetables, as you might experience issues with your digestive system if you have too many without easing your body into it. Refrain from consuming dried fruit or fruit juices as these are very high in sugar, and may cause your blood sugar to spike.

Keep your fluid intake at 64 ounces daily. This should be non-caloric beverages, and <u>as much as possible,</u> stick to water.

What shouldn't you eat after your surgery? Keep away from artificial sweeteners such as aspartame and saccharin. Unfortunately, these ingredients are commonly in a lot of food, so it is always best to read the ingredients on the label. You may use other sweeteners such as monk fruit, truvia, stevia, or sucralose in place of sugar; however, always bear in mind that moderation is key.

Vitamins and Supplements

It is recommended that you take vitamins and supplements to make sure you get enough of the recommended nutrients daily. Also, there are certain vitamins that are required for, and you will be taking for life following, bariatric surgery. A probiotic, vitamin B12, iron, and calcium are supplements you are required to take; however, when it comes to iron and calcium with vitamin D3, make sure there is at least a two-hour interval when taking these two supplements. This is because iron prevents the absorption of calcium, so <u>never</u> take them at the same time, to make sure your body absorbs all the calcium in the supplement.

Also, never take your supplements in gummy form. These do not get absorbed well, do not have all the vitamins and minerals you need, and could possibly get stuck in your digestive system.

Prior to your surgery, you may take the tablet form of the vitamins, and the liquid or chewable forms up to two months post-op.

Keep a Food Journal

Whether through an app on your phone, or old school with pen and paper, keeping a food journal lets you track your eating habits so you can see a pattern and take actions towards changing these behaviors.

These are the basic information that should be in your food journal:

- The time a meal or snack was eaten
- What kind of food was eaten and the amount
- Its macronutrients and their amounts
- How many calories it contained
- Fluid intake–what it was and how many ounces was it
- Vitamins and supplements taken
- Exercise–type and duration

If you would like deeper insight into your eating habits, you may also take note of the following information:

- Levels of hunger and fullness before and after eating
- Your mood or feelings before eating
- Who you're eating with
- Where you're eating (in front of the TV, at your desk, etc.)
- Any issues you experience after eating (pain, vomiting, etc.)
- Any food intolerances observed
- Any food worth noting because it is filling and well tolerated by your body

Here is a list of food journal apps that you can download and try:

- Baritastic: This app had a fluid intake and nutrition tracker so you can easily keep track of your caloric intake. You can set alarms so the app will remind you to take your meals, vitamins, and medications. It comes with a body mass index chart and other useful information that can help you towards a healthier lifestyle. This app also has a social component and lets you connect with a community that supports people who have gone through this surgery, and it comes with further resources about bariatric surgery.

- Waterlogged: This app helps you track your water intake. The tracker is free, although you can pay for a subscription if you want an upgrade that would include graphs. What's cool about this app is that you can record your water intake just by taking photos of your cups.

- Fooducate: The goal of this app is to educate its users about the food they eat. This app can scan any barcode and show what is in your food. Users can set up the app so it will let you know of certain information such as the presence of glucose, how much sugar is in your food, the amount of protein, etc. This information comes in handy when you're trying to consume more or avoid a specific ingredient.

- My Diet Coach: The goal of this app is to help its users maintain consistent weight loss post-surgery and in the future. You may set your goals on the app, and the My Diet Coach can help keep track of your physical activity level and caloric intake. This app provides tips for weight loss, motivational quotes, photos to inspire your weight loss journey, and a visual weight tracker.

- Happy Scale: This is the simplest app out of all five on this list. Users input their goal weight and current weight, and Happy Scale will show you a graph that has your weight loss over time.

Listen to Your Body

Be Mindful of Your Eating

Part of tracking and being aware of your eating habits is to measure how much you've eaten. Before eating, weigh and measure your food. Being more mindful of your food intake lets you be more aware of your behavior and make changes. This means:

- Eating food that nourishes, energizes, satiates, and satisfies you and your body.
- Knowing when you are hungry and when you are full.
- Not using food to deal with your issues.
- Knowing your emotional triggers that lead to emotional eating.
- Recognizing what your non-hunger triggers are that cause you to eat.
- Paying attention to your eating and eating with intention.

How can you be more mindful when eating?

- Don't feel the need to clean your plate. Listen to your body cues. When your body says you're full, stop eating even if there's still food on your plate.

- Make it a point to sit when you eat. This does not include sitting in the car and eating while driving. The purpose of sitting while eating is so you can take your time to eat and be mindful of each bite you take.

- Make a sign that says "Eat Slowly" and post it somewhere visible to you. It is easy to slip back to old habits. The sign will be a constant reminder for you to change your behavior until it becomes a habit.

- Make sure there are no distractions when you eat. There is no TV, cellphone, or computer that will keep you distracted from paying attention to each bite you take. Pick a spot in the house or work that you can go to just to eat and nothing else.

- After each bite of food you take, set your utensils down, and chew your food slowly and thoroughly.

- Take your time eating. Pay attention to each bite you take. Savor the smell of the food, the flavors, consistency, and texture.

- Take small, dime-sized bites, and chew your food at least 25 times.

- Aside from the food you're eating, pay attention to how you're feeling when you eat.

- Make your meals last at least 20 minutes. After 20 minutes, assess your hunger level and check if you're still hungry, or if you're full and can stop eating.

- Make meals a leisurely, enjoyable activity, not one that you just rush through. Set the table and use nice dishes and a placemat. Slow down and enjoy your time, and savor each bite.
- Eat your proteins first, as protein fills you up faster. When done with the proteins, move on to your vegetables.

Listen To Your Body's Hunger and Fullness Cues

Many chronic dieters have already taught themselves to ignore their body's hunger and fullness cues, and to do that, they often pick up habits such as drinking a diet soda or smoking to quell their hunger. And when it's time to eat, because they have deprived themselves, they feel the need to clean their plates even when they're already full, or worse, they overeat. Some use food to deal with stress, sadness, or boredom. Your ultimate goal is to determine your body's hunger cues and know when you're full so you can stop eating. Before eating, close your eyes, take deep breaths, and listen to your body.

Make it a habit to rate your hunger on a scale of 1 to 10, and over time, you will learn to listen to your body's cues (*Bariatric Nutrition and Lifestyle Plan*, 2017).

1	Completely empty; feeling dizzy and weak; starving
2	Stomach is growling; very hungry; irritable and low energy
3	Stomach is starting to growl; pretty hungry
4	Starting to feel hungry

5	Neither hungry nor full
6	Slightly full
7	A little uncomfortable from being full
8	Stuffed
9	Getting stomach aches from being too full
10	Nausea from being full

Ideally, you'll eat when you're feeling at around level 3 or 4. Any lower than that, and you are too hungry and risk overeating.

Take the time to get to know your body. Being full can vary from not being hungry to being in pain from eating too much, so it's important to give it your full attention. You won't be able to listen if you're distracted with work, or the TV, or driving. Use this scale every time you eat to gauge your hunger levels before you eat, while eating, and after eating.

Be More Aware of Your Body

Most people push themselves beyond their limits, working 12 to 14 hours every day, ignoring their hunger, or overeating. Most have let their mind rule over their behavior and no longer have the capability to listen to the signals their bodies give them. Your body will always tell you what it needs, though, so learn how to listen to it to keep it happy and healthy.

Physical Activity, Rest, and Dealing With Stress

Physical Activity

Exercise is as important as a healthy diet to lose weight and keep it off. Aside from the weight loss advantage, exercise also provides the following benefits:

- Helps reduce and relieve stress
- Increases your life expectancy
- Reduces your cholesterol levels
- Burns calories
- Improves your balance
- Burns fat and builds muscles
- Helps increase your energy
- Aids in weight management
- Improves sleep quality
- Lowers your blood pressure
- Helps build stronger muscles and bones
- Improves your mood

- Helps control your hunger
- Improves blood sugar levels
- Improves insulin levels

Before starting any exercise regimen, however, make sure to consult with your doctor first.

To make exercise more doable, take small steps towards getting fit. Start off with just 10 minutes of any type of physical activity. When 10 minutes is up, and you want to do another 10, go for it. If not, congratulate yourself for achieving your goal. For someone starting out with exercise, walking is the easiest form of exercise you can do. No fancy equipment needed, just get outside and start walking. If you have physical limitations on your lower body, you may also exercise while seated. There are several seated exercise videos you can follow on YouTube. Another option is to purchase an upper body ergometer, sometimes known as an arm bike, to get your exercise in while seated.

Once you've started getting into the groove of exercising and being more active, it is also important to incorporate flexibility and strength training. Strength training will help you build muscles, burn more calories, and improve your balance. Do strength training exercises for at least three times a week.

Stretching not only helps you relax and unwind, but it can also improve any problems with your balance, lengthen your muscles, and prevent injuries and back pain. A popular form of stretching is yoga.

Be mindful of your body when you exercise, especially if you experience pain in your joints. Joint pain can lead to injury, so if you experience this while exercising, modify the exercise so as not to put any further stress on that joint.

Aside from setting aside time for exercise, incorporate being more active in your daily activities. Park further away from the entrance, take the stairs instead of the elevator, take stretching breaks in front of your desk every few minutes. All these little adjustments to your routine add up to a healthier you down the road.

Sleep

Getting enough sleep is an important cornerstone in having good health and well-being. Making sure you get enough rest helps your safety, quality of living, and mental and physical health. Sufficient sleep:

- Helps improve cardiovascular health
- Boosts your immune system
- Lowers blood pressure
- Lowers stress hormones that are released into your system
- Controls your appetite and weight
- Lowers pain
- Helps make your blood sugar more manageable
- Gives you quicker reflexes
- Enhances your memory
- Improves your mood

- Allows you to think more clearly
- Boosts your focus and creativity
- Lowers your risk of injury

Target getting at least 7 hours of sleep every night, and if you feel you need more, work that into your schedule.

Regularly not getting enough sleep has long-term adverse effects on your health such as:

- Early mortality
- Diabetes
- Heart disease
- Obesity
- High blood pressure

For those who have trouble falling asleep, here are a few tips to help you catch some zzzzs:

- For better sleep, keep your bedroom cool and dark
- Eliminate nicotine, caffeine, and alcohol. These are known to disrupt sleep.
- Light from electronic devices such as tablets, mobile phones, and TV can prevent you from falling asleep, as light tricks your mind into staying awake.
- Exercise early in the day to help you sleep better. Try to avoid exercising before bedtime as the adrenaline boost can prevent you from falling asleep.
- Stick to a sleep routine that can help you relax before bedtime: Take a shower or bath, meditate, or read a book.

Managing Stress

Stress is an everyday experience for most of us. Being under constant stress affects your body in different ways:

- Brain: Stress can cause mind fog, difficulty in concentrating, moodiness, anxiety, irritability, and depression.
- Skin, Hair, and Nails: Stress can cause delayed tissue repair, hair loss, acne, dull/brittle hair, dry skin, and brittle nails.
- Cardiovascular: Stress increases your chances of getting a stroke and heart attack, increases your cholesterol level, and increases your blood pressure.
- Joints and muscles: Stress can cause your muscles to tighten, as well as cause an increase in inflammation, muscle and joint aches and pains, and muscle tension.
- Gut: Stress can cause pain and discomfort in your gut, as well as problems with nutrient absorption, bloating, diarrhea, indigestion, diarrhea, and constipation.
- Immune system: Stress can cause an increase in your recovery time from ailments, a decrease in immune function, an increased risk in becoming ill, and lowered immune defenses.
- Reproductive system: Stress can cause an increase in PMS symptoms, a decrease in hormone production, and a decrease in libido.

But the negative effects don't stop there. Stress can also affect your behavior, mind, emotions, and body in the following ways:

- Confidence loss
- Overeating
- Alienation and irritability
- Eating more high fat or high calorie food
- Depression
- Increase in alcohol consumption
- Apathy
- Lack of exercise
- Impaired judgement
- Headaches
- Negativity
- Fatigue
- Indecision
- Tight muscles
- Worrying
- Insomnia
- Restlessness
- Nightmares

These effects could hinder your path towards your weight loss goals, so it is imperative you learn how to manage your stress in healthy and effective ways. Here are a few suggestions:

- Try breaking the negativity you're experiencing that is causing you stress through prayer or meditation

- Take long, slow deep breaths
- Read a book
- Hug your loved ones or pets
- Go for a walk
- Enjoy nature
- When in a stressful situation, walk away and cool off for a few minutes
- Gardening
- Vent to a friend
- Take a nap
- Take a long hot bath or shower
- Blow bubbles

Tracking Your Progress

Measurements and Photos

It is important to take photos and measurements of your body prior to surgery and on regular intervals post-surgery. The scale weighs everything and will not always show your progress. The photos and measurements are there to provide you with visuals and evidence of your weight-loss success. Take full length front- and side-view photos and measure your hips, waist, and chest every month.

Before your surgery, choose one outfit that you can use for your "Before" photo. Each month post-op, take two photos of yourself: one wearing the "Before" outfit, and another wearing an outfit that fits you. Place these photos in a visible place, so everyday you have a reminder of your weight loss success and keep you on track with your goals.

You will need to make more effort with clothing; you need to go through your closet and sort your clothing according to size. Keep the next smaller sizes accessible, as you will lose weight very quickly after surgery. Donate the clothes that become too big for you. Do <u>not</u> enter the mindset of keeping these articles of clothing "just in case I gain weight." That should not be an option in your mind.

Changes in Your Home

Prepping Your Home

Since a lifestyle change is expected after your surgery, you need to make sure your home will help you be successful in your weight loss journey. Throw out junk food, processed food, and food with added sugars, and stock up on healthy food such as protein drinks, lean proteins, vegetables, and fruits.

Make fruits and vegetables accessible for yourself, Place them in visible areas of your house, such as placing fruits in a fruit bowl, or cutting up vegetables and placing them in a clear container in your fridge so that you reach for them when you need a snack.

If you share your home with others and they eat unhealthy food, ask them to keep their food in an area that is out of sight and not accessible to you. Try to keep your home as temptation-free as possible.

During meals, use smaller plates, and keep the food on the stove, not on the table, so that you will need to walk to the stove to refill your plate. Store leftovers immediately after eating, or throw out the food.

Keep the food weighing scale, protein shakes, blender, and other gadgets you will be using post-surgery on the kitchen counter or somewhere easy to access so they are visible to you and act as a reminder for you to use.

Shopping for Food

When shopping for food, always make a grocery list and stick to it. Keep the lean proteins, fruits, and vegetables at the top of the list.

Make sure that you eat prior to going to the grocery store. Most people have a tendency to pick up extra, unhealthy items if they're food shopping when hungry.

Once at the supermarket, try to avoid the middle aisles, which is where most stores keep their processed and junk foods. The whole food can usually be found around the perimeter of the store.

Only buy necessities for you and your family. Don't buy unhealthy food for other people that you may eat, like cereal loaded with added sugar, for example. Don't give yourself a chance to be tempted by unhealthy food. Stock up on fruits and vegetables instead–the fresh, frozen, and canned types. While canned fruits and vegetables are less nutritious than their fresh counterparts, they are a lot healthier to eat than fast food and as convenient to access. For canned fruits, purchase the ones that are packed in their own juices, not the ones with added syrup or sugar.

Items to Purchase Pre- and Post-Surgery

- Blender
- Slow cooker
- Ice cube tray: You can freeze pre-made pureed food in these trays to consume at your convenience.
- Child-sized plates and utensils: Smaller plates and utensils can help you control your portions and slow you down when eating.
- Food scale, measuring spoons, and measuring cups: Part of being aware of what you eat, includes measuring your food intake.
- Food journal: So you can record your eating habits.
- A few high protein, low or no-sugar beverages: Do not buy too many, but do buy a variety. Some people experience their tastes and preferences changing after their surgery.
- Other sugar-free, non-caffeinated, non-carbonated beverages: Flavored water or decaffeinated herbal tea, for example.

- Sucralose to add to your protein shakes, if needed.

- Herbs and spices: To enhance the flavor of your food. Just stay away from the spicy seasoning, as spicy food might cause an adverse reaction in your digestive system.

- Vitamins and supplements: Buy a few of the tablet form for pre-surgery consumption, and the liquid or chewable forms for the first two months after your surgery.

Your Support System

Family and Friends

It is important to have a strong support system with family and friends for those who have suffered from obesity and have gone through gastric sleeve surgery. Your support system can help keep you on track when old habits manifest itself. Let your support system know how they can best support your weight loss journey. Do you need your spouse to watch the kids while you take an hour or two to exercise? Do you need everyone in your household to help you keep forbidden food hidden or inaccessible? Have a conversation with them so they also know what they can do to help. You, on the other hand, must also be willing to receive the help.

Have someone from your support group attend one of your medical appointments or a support group meeting so they are aware of the process.

Aside from family and friends, it would be beneficial to find exercise buddies. It's harder to give up exercising if you have someone to exercise with.

Bariatric Medical Team

Your Bariatric Medical Team is also another important support system you will have. Make sure you keep all of your bariatric medical appointments to ensure you are on top of any changes in your nutritional and medical needs. The follow up check ups could be with your dietitian, surgeon, nurse, or the physician assistant. During your consultation, an assessment will be made to see if you are adjusting as you should be to the surgery; your food intake will be reviewed to make sure you're maximizing your weight loss, and they will go over your weight loss progress. They will also discuss with you any possible complications you may experience from the surgery or from your behavior. They will check in with you on the status of your other health conditions, if applicable, and adjust your medications if needed. You will also have lab tests done, and they will go over the results.

Attending your post-op sessions with your medical team is important so that any problems that come up over time can be addressed.

Before meeting with your Bariatric Medical Team, make sure to prepare beforehand. Write down any questions you have and discuss with them during your session. Have your food records ready and totaled. Have the information to the following questions ready:

- Do you have problems grazing?
- Are you experiencing vomiting, nausea, or other issues?
- Are you staying full?
- How much is your average daily consumption of protein in grams?
- Which sources are you getting your protein from?
- Are you exercising? If so, what type of exercise(s) are you doing, the duration, and the frequency in a week?
- On average, how many calories do you consume in a day?
- Which vitamins and supplements are you taking and in what forms?
- How much is your average daily fluid intake?
- Are you consuming your fluids separately from your meals? How many minutes before and after each meal?

You can get support from your Bariatric Nutritionist for all questions regarding food and nutrition. They are there to educate and support you so your weight loss is maximized and nutrition is optimized. Since the surgery alters your body, your nutritional needs change dramatically compared to before your surgery. You will need to change your eating habits and adopt new ones. Your dietician can help you create meal plans that can meet your nutritional needs.

There will be several sessions with your dietitian. The first one will be before your surgery. Your dietitian will discuss the various diet stages before and after surgery. They will discuss how to make your new lifestyle as enjoyable and successful as possible, create meal plans for you, and answer any questions you may have about diet and nutrition.

The second session will be held about a week after your surgery. In this session, your dietician will review your current progress, help you create meal plans for the upcoming phases, and answer any more questions you may have about your diet and nutrition.

Two months after your surgery, you will meet with your dietician again. They will go over your progress and make any adjustments to your meal plans so you can meet your nutritional needs and maximize weight loss. They will also be available to answer any questions you may have.

Six months after your surgery, you will have another meeting with your dietician to again, review your progress and answer any questions you may have. They will then help you make meal plans to meet your nutritional needs.

You may continue to have sessions with your dietitian from time to time to check in on your progress, or if you need to discuss any adjustments to your plans that you may need.

Part 2

Introduction

Chapter 1: Understanding Gastric Sleeve Surgery

- **What is Gastric Sleeve Surgery**

Vertical sleeve gastrectomy, also known as the gastric sleeve surgery is a process in which the stomach's capacity to hold the food is reduced by 80 percent. IN other words, a sleeve is created on the side of the stomach, which receives the food in a small amount; the rest is separated through this surgery. This bariatric procedure is also called weight loss surgery as it is used to induce weight loss through a permanent approach. The following diagram shows how the stomach walls are stitched together to create a separate sleeve for food digestion:

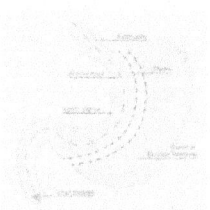

Diagram: Post Gastric Sleeve Surgery Stomach

- **Why is It Needed?**

The gastric sleeve surgery is mainly opted to achieve weight loss. This surgery works for people who are sensitive to dietary changes and just can't lose weight through diet control. So, this surgery finds a permanent solution and reduces the stomach size, which automatically cuts down the food consumption.

This surgery has given effective results, and within one year of the surgery, people should 70 percent weight loss. By controlling obesity, such individuals were also able to resist diabetes, insulin resistance, sleep apnea, hypertension, joints pain, fatty liver disease, and hyperlipidemia. Excessive hunger sensation is also reduced to a minimum after gastric sleeve surgery. The procedure is indeed effective, but it works well only when a person changes his dietary habits after the surgery and follows a gastric sleeve diet.

- **Pre-Surgery Tips**
1. Change your diet and switch to liquid-only diet a week before the surgery.
2. If you are a smoker, then stop smoking at least 2 weeks before the surgery to avoid complications.
3. Discuss your health condition and post-surgery effects with your doctor before the surgery.
4. Clean your kitchen and set up the pantry according to the new lifestyle.
5. Increase the protein intake to prepare the body for quick recovery after the surgery.

- **Post-Surgery Tips:**
1. Switch to the gastric sleeve diet and use more clear liquids right after the surgery.
2. Add protein-based supplements and liquids to the diet to ensure quick recovery and healing of the stomach.
3. Start with the intake of soft food and gradually switch to the proper meals.
4. Stop having heavy, oily food on the table.
5. Light exercises and yoga ensure quick recovery, so try some light exercises 2-3 days after the surgery.
6. Consult your dietician and the doctor after every week to discuss your diet and changing health conditions.

Chapter 2: Gastric Sleeve Diet

- **What to have on the Gastric Sleeve diet?**

It is important to notice here that the gastric sleeve diet plan must be planned according to the post-op healing process. It takes 4 weeks to recover and adjust the body after the gastric sleeve surgery. The food on this diet is, therefore divided according to the five stages:

1. First week: This week is the week of clear liquids only, and the person must only take light liquids like broths, unsweetened juices, decaffeinated drinks, etc.
2. Second Week: In this, a person may start taking food in the form of purees that can be easily digested by the stomach. The dieter can consume:

- instant breakfast drinks
- nonfat, sugar-free, pudding
- shakes made with protein powder
- thin broth and cream soups
- unsweetened milk
- sugar-free, nonfat frozen, ice cream, yogurt and sorbet
- nonfat plain Greek yogurt
- fruit juices with no pulp, diluted with water
- thinned, hot cereal, such as oatmeal or Cream of Wheat

3. Third Week: In this week, a person can start taking proper food but in a soft or semi-solid form, such as follows:
   - cooked, pureed white fish
   - soft-scrambled or soft-boiled eggs
   - silken tofu
   - soup
   - cottage cheese
   - canned fruit in juice
   - hummus
   - pureed or mashed avocado
   - mashed bananas or very ripe mango
   - plain Greek yogurt

4. Fourth week: by the start of this week, the stomach is almost healed so it can digest food easily. So, the dieter can eat following items easily:
   - well-cooked chicken and fish
   - well-cooked vegetables
   - sweet potatoes
   - low-fat cheese
   - fruit
   - low-sugar cereal
   - **What to avoid on a Gastric Sleeve diet?**

Since the stomach size is reduced after the surgery, a person avoids all such things that would occupy the stomach space without providing healthy energy.

Following things must be avoided on the gastric sleeve diet:

1. Eating and drinking at the same time.
2. Sugary products and beverages.
3. Alcohol-based drinks.
4. Saturate fats and products containing such fats.
5. Bread, rice, and pasta
6. Highly caffeinated drinks
7. Dry food items
8. Tough meats like beef steak, chops, hot dogs and ham, etc.
9. Anti-inflammatory drugs like ibuprofen, naproxen, and aspirin.

- **What to have on the Gastric Sleeve diet?**

It is important to notice here that the gastric sleeve diet plan must be planned according to the post-op healing process. It takes 4 weeks to recover and adjust the body after the gastric sleeve surgery. The food on this diet is, therefore divided according to the five stages:

5. First week: This week is the week of clear liquids only, and the person must only take light liquids like broths, unsweetened juices, decaffeinated drinks, etc.
6. Second Week: In this, a person may start taking food in the form of purees that can be easily digested by the stomach. The dieter can consume:

- instant breakfast drinks
- nonfat, sugar-free, pudding

- shakes made with protein powder
- thin broth and cream soups
- unsweetened milk
- sugar-free, nonfat frozen, ice cream, yogurt and sorbet
- nonfat plain Greek yogurt
- fruit juices with no pulp, diluted with water
- thinned, hot cereal, such as oatmeal or Cream of Wheat

7. Third Week: In this week, a person can start taking proper food but in a soft or semi-solid form, such as follows:
- cooked, pureed white fish
- soft-scrambled or soft-boiled eggs
- silken tofu
- soup
- cottage cheese
- canned fruit in juice
- hummus
- pureed or mashed avocado
- mashed bananas or very ripe mango
- plain Greek yogurt

8. Fourth week: by the start of this week, the stomach is almost healed so it can digest food easily. So, the dieter can eat following items easily:
- well-cooked chicken and fish
- well-cooked vegetables

- sweet potatoes
- low-fat cheese
- fruit
- low-sugar cereal
- **What to avoid on a Gastric Sleeve diet?**

Since the stomach size is reduced after the surgery, a person avoids all such things that would occupy the stomach space without providing healthy energy. Following things must be avoided on the gastric sleeve diet:

10. Eating and drinking at the same time.
11. Sugary products and beverages.
12. Alcohol-based drinks.
13. Saturate fats and products containing such fats.
14. Bread, rice, and pasta
15. Highly caffeinated drinks
16. Dry food items
17. Tough meats like beef steak, chops, hot dogs and ham, etc.
18. Anti-inflammatory drugs like ibuprofen, naproxen, and aspirin.

Chapter 3: The Clear Liquids Diet

A clear liquid diet is recommended on the post-op stage after the gastric sleeve surgery. It is mainly because that few days after the surgery, the healing phase initiates, and the stomach isn't capable of processes nutrients and calories in the food, but the body does need hydration. Clear liquid provides much-needed minerals, metabolites, and moisture that the body needs; therefore, they are given to a person after the surgery for a quick recovery. The following are the clear liquids that must be consumed on the bariatric diet.

1. Broth
2. Unsweetened juice
3. Decaffeinated tea or coffee
4. Milk (skim or 1 percent)
5. Sugar-free gelatine drinks

Gastric Sleeve Diet Recipes

Chapter 4: Breakfast Recipes

Strawberry & Yogurt Smoothie Bowl

Yield: 2 servings

Preparation Time: 15 minutes

Total Time: 15 minutes

Ingredients:

- 2 cups frozen strawberries
- ½ cup unsweetened almond milk
- ¼ cup fat-free plain Greek yogurt
- 1 tablespoon unsweetened whey protein powder
- 3 tablespoons fresh strawberries, hulled and sliced
- 2 tablespoons walnuts, chopped

Instructions:

1. In a blender, add frozen strawberries and pulse for about 1 minute.
2. Add the almond milk, yogurt and protein powder and pulse until desired consistency is achieved.
3. Divide the smoothie mixture into 2 serving bowls evenly.

4. Serve immediately with the topping of strawberry slices and walnuts.

Blueberry & Veggies Smoothie Bowl

Yield: 3 servings

Preparation Time: 15 minutes

Total Time: 15 minutes

Ingredients:

- 1 cup frozen blueberries
- 1½ cups frozen spinach leaves
- ½ cup zucchini, chopped roughly
- ½ cup cauliflower florets, chopped roughly
- 1¼ cups unsweetened almond milk
- 3 tablespoons hemp hearts
- 2 tablespoons almond butter
- 1 teaspoon ground cinnamon
- 1 teaspoon vanilla extract
- 2-3 drops liquid stevia
- 1 banana, peeled and sliced

Instructions:

1. Add all ingredients in a high-speed blender except for banana slices and pulse until smooth.
2. Transfer the mixture into 3 serving bowls evenly.
3. Top with banana slices and serve immediately.

Warm Fruity & Cheese Bowl

Yield: 2 servings

Preparation Time: 15 minutes

Cooking Time: 8 minutes

Total Time: 23 minutes

Ingredients:

- 1 Granny Smith apple, peeled, cored and chopped
- ½ cup frozen unsweetened cherries
- 1 teaspoon pure maple syrup
- 2 tablespoons freshly squeezed lemon juice
- 2-3 tablespoons filtered water
- 1 cup fresh raspberries
- ½ teaspoon fresh orange zest, grated finely
- ½ teaspoon ground cinnamon
- 1 teaspoon vanilla extract
- 1½ cups low-fat cottage cheese
- 3 tablespoons almonds, toasted and chopped

Instructions:

1. In a pan, add the apple, cherries, maple syrup, lemon juice and water and stir to combine.
2. Now, place the pan over medium heat and cook until boiling, stirring occasionally.

3. Add the raspberries, orange zest and spices and stir to combine.
4. Degrease the heat to low and simmer, covered for about 5-8 minutes, stirring occasionally.
5. Remove from the heat and immediately, stir in the vanilla extract.
6. Cover the pan and set aside for about 10 minutes.
7. Uncover the pan and stir the mixture well.
8. Set aside for about 10 minutes.
9. Meanwhile, in a bowl, add the cottage cheese and almonds and mix well.
10. Divide the cheese mixture in 2 serving bowls.
11. Top with warm fruity mixture and serve.

Cheese & Yogurt Bowl

Yield: 2 servings

Preparation Time: 15 minutes

Cooking Time: 8 minutes

Total Time: 23 minutes

Ingredients:

- ½ cup plain fat-free Greek yogurt
- ½ cup low-fat cottage cheese
- 2 teaspoons extra-virgin olive oil
- ¼ teaspoon ground cinnamon
- 2 medium apples, cored and cubed
- ½ cup fresh blackberries
- ½ cup fresh blueberries
- ¼ cup walnuts, chopped

Instructions:

1. In a large bowl, add the yogurt, cheese, oil and cinnamon and mix until well combined.
2. Gently, fold in the apple and berries.
3. Divide the yogurt mixture in 2 serving bowls.
4. Top with walnuts and serve *immediately*.

Banana Porridge

Yield: 4 servings

Preparation Time: 10 minutes

Total Time: 10 minutes

Ingredients:

- 4 large ripe bananas, peeled, sliced and mashed
- 1 tablespoon almond butter, softened
- ½ teaspoon ground cinnamon
- ¼ cup walnuts, chopped
- ½ cup fresh blueberries

Instructions:

1. In a large bowl, place bananas, almond butter and cinnamon and stir to combine.
2. Top with walnuts and blueberries and serve.

Pumpkin Porridge

Yield: 4 servings

Preparation Time: 10 minutes

Cooking Time: 1 hour

Total Time: 1 hour 10 minutes

Ingredients:

- 1 medium pumpkin, cut in half
- 2 cups unsweetened almond milk
- 1 large banana, peeled and sliced

Instructions:

1. Preheat your oven to350 degrees F.
2. Line a baking sheet with a greased parchment paper.
3. Place the pumpkin n prepared baking sheet, cut side down.
4. Bake for about 1 hour.
5. Remove the baking sheet from oven and set aside to cool slightly.
6. Now, remove the seeds and then scoop out the inner side of pumpkin.
7. Transfer the pumpkin flesh into a bowl and with a fork, mash it completely.
8. Transfer the mashed pumpkin in serving bowls.
9. Pour milk over mashed pumpkin.

10. Top with banana slices and serve.

Overnight Banana Oatmeal

Yield: 3 servings

Preparation Time: 10 minutes

Total Time: 10 minutes

Ingredients:

- 1 cup rolled oats
- 2 bananas, peeled and mashed
- 2 tablespoons chia seeds
- 2 teaspoons matcha green tea
- 1½ cups unsweetened almond milk
- 3 tablespoons almonds, chopped

Instructions:

1. Place all ingredients except almonds in a large bowl and mix until well combined.
2. Cover the bowl and refrigerate overnight.
3. In the morning, remove the bowl from refrigerator.
4. Top with almonds and serve.

Pumpkin & Cottage Cheese Oatmeal

Yield: 1 serving

Preparation Time: 10 minutes

Cooking Time: 2½ minutes

Total Time: 12½ minutes

Ingredients:

- 1/3 cup old fashioned oats
- ½ cup canned sugar-free pumpkin
- 1 teaspoon Truvia baking blend
- 1/8 teaspoon ground cinnamon
- Pinch of ground cloves
- Pinch of ground ginger
- ½ cup no salt added 1% cottage cheese
- 1 tablespoon walnuts, chopped

Instructions:

1. In a microwave-safe bowl, add the oats, pumpkin, Truvia baking blend and spices and stir to combine.
2. Now cook in microwave on High for about 90 seconds, stirring once after 50 seconds.
3. Remove from the microwave and stir in the cottage cheese.
4. Again, microwave on High for about 60 seconds, stirring once after 30 seconds.

5. Remove from the microwave and set aside for about 2 minutes before eating.
6. Top with walnuts and serve.

Vanilla Crepes

Yield: 4 servings

Preparation Time: 10 minutes

Cooking Time: 8 minutes

Total Time: 18 minutes

Ingredients:

- 2 tablespoons arrowroot powder
- 2 tablespoons almond flour
- ½ teaspoon ground cinnamon
- 4 eggs
- 1 teaspoon vanilla extract
- Olive oil cooking spray

Instructions:

1. In a bowl, add the arrowroot powder, almond flour and cinnamon and mix well.
2. In another bowl, add the eggs and vanilla extract and beat until well combined.
3. Add the egg mixture into the bowl of flour mixture and mix until well combined.
4. Lightly, grease a large non-stick skillet with cooking spray and heat over medium-high heat.
5. Add the desired amount of mixture and tilt the pan to spread in an even and thin layer.

6. Cook for 1 minute or until bottom becomes golden brown.
7. Carefully, flip the side and cook for about 1 minute more or until golden brown.
8. Repeat with the remaining mixture.
9. Serve warm.

www.ingramcontent.com/pod-product-compliance
Lightning Source LLC
Chambersburg PA
CBHW071437070526
44578CB00001B/109